IDENTIFYING HANDICAPPED CHILDREN: a guide to casefinding, screening, diagnosis, assessment, and evaluation, ed. by Lee Cross and Kennith W. Goin. Walker & Co., for the Technical Assistance Development System, a div. of the Frank Porter Graham Child Development Center at the University of North Carolina at Chapel Hill, 1977. 127p ill bibl index 76-52246. 8.95 ISBN 0-8027-9041-0; 6.95 pa ISBN 0-8027-7111-4

Well written, nicely organized, and well edited, this compilation is divided into two major parts. Part I is divided into five chapters that provide an excellent conceptual framework and review the structure of an ideal identification program and its five components: casefinding; screening; diagnosis; educational assessment; and program evaluation. This little volume is a good starting point for undergraduates and others who need to understand the scope of identification services for exceptional children. Chapter 1 discusses casefinding procedures and defines the target population as children from birth to eight years of age. In the second chapter, there is a good rationale for screening and the difference between screening and differential diagnosis tactics. The chapter on differential diagnosis identifies many sources of error. Chapter 4 distinguishes between norm-referenced and criterion-referenced tests, and discusses their use, strengths, and weaknesses and gives some excellent examples. In Part II there is a very good alphabetical, annotated, test bibliography that is keyed to the kind of test and the curriculum area surveyed.

IDENTIFYING
HANDICAPPED
CHILDREN

IDENTIFYING HANDICAPPED CHILDREN:
A Guide to Casefinding, Screening, Diagnosis, Assessment and Evaluation

edited by Lee Cross and Kennith W. Goin

119343

Published by

 WALKER AND COMPANY
720 Fifth Avenue
New York, NY 10019

for

The Technical Assistance Development System
A Division of Frank Porter Graham
Child Development Center at
The University of North Carolina, Chapel Hill

This book was developed pursuant to a grant from the United States Office of Education. Grantees who undertake such projects under government sponsorship are encouraged to express freely their judgment in professional and technical matters. Points of view or opinions do not, therefore, necessarily represent official Office of Education position or policy.

First published in the United States of America in 1977 by the Walker Publishing Company, Inc.

Published simultaneously in Canada by Fitzhenry & Whiteside, Limited, Toronto

CLOTH ISBN: 0-8027-9041-0
PAPER ISBN: 0-8027-7111-4

Library of Congress Catalog Card Number: 76-52246

Printed in the United States of America

10 9 8 7 6 5 4 3 2 1

Contents

Foreword vii

PART ONE—A GUIDE TO CASEFINDING, SCREENING, DIAGNOSIS, ASSESSMENT AND EVALUATION 1

CHAPTER 1   An Introduction *Lee Cross* 3

CHAPTER 2   Casefinding *Lee Cross* 9

CHAPTER 3   Screening *David L. Lillie* 17

CHAPTER 4   Diagnosis *Art Cross* 25

CHAPTER 5   Educational Assessment *Gloria Harbin* 35

CHAPTER 6   Program Evaluation *Melvin G. Moore* 53

PART TWO—A BIBLIOGRAPHY OF SCREENING, DIAGNOSIS AND ASSESSMENT INSTRUMENTS 59

CHAPTER 7   Introduction *Lee Cross* 61

CHAPTER 8   The Bibliography *Lee Cross and Sonya Johnston* 63

CHAPTER 9   The Matrix: A Guide to the Instruments *Lee Cross* 111

Index 123

Foreword

When this book was begun in 1975, the confusion surrounding the processes involved in locating children who have remediable handicaps and preparing programs to ameliorate their conditions was at its peak. In that year, Congress passed Public Law 94-142 or *The Education for All Handicapped Children Acts of 1975.* This law stipulated that each state had to develop a plan for identifying, locating, and evaluating all children in the state who were handicapped, and that it had to develop a "practical method for finding who is and who is not (being) served" under existing services. In essence, this Act meant that all states wanting federal support for their handicapped children would have to develop identification programs that were far more sophisticated, both in terms of structure and the number of people they served, than present efforts.

This book was developed to guide educators at state and local administration levels who wish to develop programs for serving handicapped children. While their design may vary, all effective programs must contain certain basic elements. Five elements— casefinding, screening, diagnosis, educational assessment, and program evaluation—are necessary for programs to serve the needs of clients *comprehensively.* Through IDENTIFYING HANDICAPPED CHILDREN, we have tried to alleviate much of the confusion which surrounds the use and definition of these five activities.

Part I of this book defines the scope of an identification program and examines the five elements. Chapter 1 reviews the structure of an ideal program and briefly describes the relationships between the various elements in the structure, while Chapters 2-6 offer detailed discussions of each of the major elements. Part II of the book is an annotated bibliography of screening, diagnosis, and assessment devices. It includes information on prices and availability of listed materials.

The content of this book is intended to be a starting point for those who wish to understand the scope of identification services for children and for those who face the enormous task of designing and/or implementing identification services. We trust that it will prove useful to all who are working to serve handicapped children.

PART ONE

A Guide to Casefinding, Screening, Diagnosis, Assessment and Evaluation

CHAPTER *1*

An Introduction
Lee Cross

This book is designed to address the needs of those involved in planning and implementing "child identification" programs. These programs may include providing appropriate placement, developing individual program plans, and providing appropriate educational activities for young handicapped children. The chapters in this book provide a conceptual framework for developing a sound identification program, which includes casefinding, screening, diagnostic, educational assessment, and program evaluation services. The procedures which are addressed are relevant to state and local education agency staffs, as well as to the staffs of single programs. The services are similar even though they may take place at various levels within a state.

The planning and implementation of *casefinding, screening,* and *diagnostic* services may occur at the state level, and the state may be directly responsible for the provision of each service. Or, the services may be planned by a state education agency but be implemented by local agencies. *Educational assessment* and *program evaluation,* on the other hand, are for the most part the responsibility of the local program staff. The state education agency, however, may be responsible for the development of guidelines.

This book is divided into two main sections. Part I is composed of five chapters. Each of the chapters includes a definition of its topic, an explanation of purposes, and a discussion of the procedures which may be used in implementing the activity. Part II, an annotated bibliography of instruments, provides information on the screening, diagnostic, and assessment instruments appropriate

LEE CROSS is Director of Early Childhood Education at the Frank Porter Graham Child Development Center at the University of North Carolina, Chapel Hill. Her interests include programming for preschool handicapped children and assessment.

for children, ages birth through eight. The first part is designed to introduce the reader to the scope of the activities outlined in Figure 1, while the second part is intended to provide a guide to the material resources available.

The five activities covered in this book are very closely related and, in some cases, overlap. The following discussion has been included in this chapter to familiarize the reader with the relationships between the activities and the nature of each particular activity.

Casefinding is a systematic process for locating handicapped or potentially handicapped children who will profit from early intervention services. Casefinding may be those procedures involved in locating children for screening or diagnostic activities, depending on the program's goals and objectives. The casefinding process includes defining the target population, increasing the public's awareness of services, encouraging referrals, and canvassing the community for children in need of services.

The casefinding procedures selected by a program depend on the nature of the target population. For example, a project serving newborn to two-year-old physically handicapped children within a fifty-mile radius might only need to contact all pediatricians and newborn care units in hospitals within fifty miles. Whereas a project whose target populations is three- to five-year-old children with mild mental handicaps will undoubtedly have to advertise services, encourage referrals from social service and health agencies, and canvass neighborhoods.

Information gained during casefinding may simplify the screening process considerably. The number of children located to participate in screening is dependent on the thoroughness of the casefinding procedures. It is quite clear that if the goal is to find a large number of children to participate in screening, casefinding must involve more than a public awareness program.

Screening is a measurement activity which identifies in the general population those children that appear to be in need of special services in order to develop to their maximum potential. The intent of screening is to review a large number of children for a particular handicap or deviance in development in a fast and efficient way. For example, in Smith County there are 1,000 children between three and five years of age. If the goal of the program is to identify and provide services to all county children with delays in two or more developmental areas, the most efficient and economical first step in the identification process would be to screen all three- to five-year-old children in the county to find those with possible developmental delays. On the other hand, if the goal

FIGURE 1

An Overview

ACTIVITY	PURPOSE	WHO
CASE-FINDING	To Make Initial Contact With Target Population And Increase The Public's Awareness of Services	Program Staff, Volunteers, Community Members
SCREENING	To Sort Out Children Needing Further Study	Volunteers, Professionals, Paraprofessionals
DIAGNOSIS	To Determine Extent Of Medical And Developmental/Educational Impairments	Psychologist, Speech and Language Therapist, Pediatrician, Neurologist, Social Worker, Nurse
	To Determine Treatment And Program Placement	
EDUCATIONAL ASSESSMENT	To Determine Individual Objectives, Strategies and Inter-Treatment (Curriculum) Activities	Teachers, Parents
PROGRAM EVALUATION	To Determine Effectiveness of Program	Program Staff, Evaluation Consultant

is to identify and provide services to all three- to five-year-old cerebral palsied children, this countywide screening would probably not be the most appropriate procedure to use, since it would be time-consuming and expensive. In most cases, it is not necessary to screen for severe handicaps, because this population can be identified during casefinding.

Screening is a source of valuable information about the development of children, but it has its limitations in that it can only indicate the possible presence of an impairment. Therefore, children should not be labeled on the basis of screening, and intervention should not be determined or planned without diagnostic study. Screening should provide project staff with enough information about a child to decide: (1) if he is a candidate for thorough diagnostic study, or (2) if he has a good prognosis for success without receiving special services. Screening should take place only if appropriate diagnostic and program services are available. If such services are unavailable, the costs in time and money expended for screening activities and the unnecessary anxiety created in the parents of the children identified for further examination make screening unjustifiable.

Frequently, parent questionnaires are coupled with screening instruments to aid in the identification process. Parents are extremely good observers of their own children, and they have little difficulty in sharing their observations when the questions directed to them deal with the child's usual daily activities. On the other hand, questions which deal with activities which are unusual or infrequent bring less reliable responses.

The purpose of the screening program and the procedures to be used therein should be explained to the parents, as should the results of the screening and their implications for further testing. In cases where a child fails the screening, the parents should be made aware that the child needs further diagnosis before any conclusive decisions can be made about his suspected condition.

Thorough screening will help avoid expensive and time-consuming diagnostic procedures for those who will not benefit from early intervention. In addition, information gained in screening should help facilitate the diagnostic process in that screening should indicate the strengths and weaknesses of a child. The screening process may be limited in the case of children with severe and profound handicaps.

Diagnosis involves looking at a child and his environment in depth for four basic purposes:

1. to determine whether a handicapping condition (or conditions) exists;

2. to clarify the causes of the identified problem (i.e., is the child nonverbal due to a hearing impairment, mental retardation, an information-process problem, or lack of verbal stimulation);
3. to develop a treatment plan;
4. to ascertain the most appropriate service that the program can render the child.

Diagnosis is more specific than screening and ideally should involve a multidisciplinary team of trained professionals. The composition of this team will vary, depending on the nature of the child's disability. In determining the composition of the team, one must initially decide the type of data needed to determine the appropriate program service and treatment for the child. Data should be obtained from as many disciplines as possible in order to prepare as broad a picture as possible of the child's performance. Individuals who might be involved in the diagnosis are: a physician, a psychologist, a social worker, an educational diagnostician, a neurologist, a psychiatrist, a physical therapist, and a language therapist.

It is important that the multidisciplinary team utilize information that is already available, such as the screening results which should give direction in prescribing further evaluations. If a child passes the hearing and vision screening, for example, it would be a waste of time to do a more in-depth evaluation in these areas. However, if a child shows a delay in the language area based on screening results, it would be advantageous to have a speech and language clinician do a more in-depth examination. Diagnostic procedures are costly and time-consuming. Therefore, it is important to keep in mind that personnel should not be involved in data collection unless their expertise is genuinely warranted; i.e., it will improve the decision-making capabilities of the multidisciplinary team.

Procedures within the diagnostic phase include the administration of standardized instruments, systematic observation, development of social and case histories, and formal interviews. After the appropriate data have been obtained and analyzed, the multidisciplinary team along with the parent(s) should, as a group, synthesize and interpret the combined results in order to reach mutual agreement on the findings. A treatment plan should be developed along with recommendations for educational programming.

Once the treatment plan has been determined, appropriate services should be considered and options analyzed. It will often be necessary for supportive services as well as the educational service to be identified. It is helpful for parents if the multidisciplinary team can identify and facilitate this referral.

The information obtained from the results of the diagnostic activities should have strong implications for developing an individualized program for each child. This information should not be discarded once the child is placed in appropriate services. Results should be interpreted to staff and parents with emphasis on implications for the planning of daily activities for the child.

Educational assessment, within this context, involves those ongoing procedures during which the teacher and/or parent determines individual goals and objectives in specific areas of development in order to plan an educational program for the child. Assessment activities usually take place following diagnosis.

The outcome of the assessment process should be a profile of the individual to enable those working with the child to identify strengths as well as weaknesses. Assessment provides the teacher with a vehicle for planning a series of specific curriculum experiences that are based on specific goals and objectives related to the information derived from assessment.

Program evaluation is discussed in this work to clarify its relation to diagnosis and educational assessment. There are two essential purposes for evaluation: (1) to collect data and information on the program for internal decision making, and (2) to provide information for external agencies and populations such as consumers, the Bureau of Education for the Handicapped, and future replication sites. Evaluation as used in this book does not refer to measurement of an individual child's skills and abilities.

Ongoing evaluation activities provide teachers and parents with program data and information which demonstrate the effectiveness of instructional activities used in reaching instructional objectives. This evaluation information assists staff in planning appropriate activities for children in addition to documenting program effectiveness. Periodic rediagnostic activities by members of the multidisciplinary team can also provide staff with program evaluation information on child progress as well as new directions that need to be taken.

Evaluation activities for external audiences should produce data which demonstrate what children can do after intervention that they could not do before, or demonstrate what conditions existed before intervention that no longer exist. Examples of this kind of data would be summarized in ongoing assessment data as well as information from the periodic rediagnostic activities.

CHAPTER 2

Casefinding
Lee Cross

WHAT IS CASEFINDING?

Casefinding is a planned set of procedures whereby children are systematically located for screening. Casefinding is not the application of any instrument; it is the first step in the identification process during which names are obtained for screening. During casefinding, parents and the community are informed of the services (screening, diagnosis, and intervention) that are or will be available.

WHY IS IT IMPORTANT TO BE AWARE OF THE TARGET POPULATION?

Before children can be located for screening, it is essential to know the target population that is to receive services. This knowledge will help in avoiding overrecruitment of children and in selecting appropriate casefinding strategies. The following characteristics of the target population need to be considered in the selection of appropriate and effective casefinding procedures: (1) the age range to be served; (2) the handicapping condition for which intervention services are available; and (3) the geographical boundaries of the population to be served.

The age range to be served. The age range in part determines the casefinding procedures that will be used. If infants are to be served, for example, it would be logical to contact pediatricians, check Apgar scores, and communicate with neonatal or high-risk clinics in hospitals within the geographical area. However, it would *not* be profitable to contact nursery schools or day-care centers serving three- to five-year-old children.

The handicapping condition to be served. The type and degree of handicap influences the selection of appropriate casefinding procedures. It is, of course, simpler to locate those children that are more severely handicapped than those mildly involved. Likewise, physical handicaps, such as deafness and blindness, are easily located if parents, caretakers, and physicians are made cognizant of these disabilities at a fairly early age. Community agency staffs and health personnel will often be aware of children with severe and profound handicaps, because the parents of such children often seek services when their child is very young. "Finding" the majority of this population often can be accomplished by contacting agencies and community workers.

If the handicap is mild or moderate, the location effort becomes more difficult. It may be necessary to locate and recruit all children within a given age range so that they can be screened for a particular handicapping condition. Efforts need to be made to find all children within the age range for screening to insure that all children with a particular handicap are found.

Geographical boundaries. The geographical boundaries in which the target population for services resides dictates the type of casefinding procedures that will be implemented. The demographic conditions within a geographical target influence the type of activities. For example, strategies within a sparsely populated rural area will be different than activities in an urban area. In addition, knowledge of the geographical boundaries limits the area in which location activities need to take place.

All characteristics of the target population must be considered in conjunction with one another in determining procedures for locating children for screening. Currently, many states are involved in the development and implementation of statewide "child find" activities that are designed to locate all three- to five-year-old handicapped children who are currently unserved. This group represents the broadest possible target population. Hopefully, states and programs will make an effort to develop comprehensive casefinding procedures *in order to find children to participate in screening, diagnostic, and intervention services*. To simply locate children without providing services is a waste of time and money.

WHAT PROCESS IS USED TO LOCATE CHILDREN?

The location of preschool (0-5) children with handicaps or potential handicaps is a unique situation. Preschool children are scattered throughout the community and are not normally found in one setting as are school-age children. The casefinding process is a combination of procedures which are determined by the characteristics of the community, the types of resources available, and the nature of the target population. The casefinding process includes developing an awareness of services, encouraging referrals, canvassing the community to recruit children, and recording names obtained from referrals, awareness activities, and the community canvass. This set of procedures is comprehensive. Consequently, all procedures need to be implemented in conjunction with one another. One procedure alone will not be effective.

WHAT IS MEANT BY PUBLIC AWARENESS ACTIVITIES?

Activities which inform the public of the existence of specific program services and the procedures whereby eligible children will be identified should be conducted on an ongoing basis. Awareness is the stage before handicapped children have been initially identified and/or before parents and the community have been informed of available program services.

Awareness activities might include using television, radio, newspaper, and other media; sending information sheets and letters to community members and parents; establishing and maintaining a toll free telephone hotline service; placing posters and leaflets in banks, grocery stores, launderettes, beauty parlors, barber shops, libraries, municipal buildings, and churches; and arranging speaking engagements at PTA's, churches, parent meetings, and civic organizations. A prime focus of awareness activities should be local service agencies, professional meetings, and the medical community—particularly pediatricians.

An effective way to involve pediatricians in the casefinding process is to gain the support of an influential member of the medical community and utilize his influence to gain the support of other members. In addition to the involvement of private pediatricians, it is essential to gain the support of public health nurses and the staffs working in clinics.

Those developing materials for public awareness should make sure that the type and nature of their presentation is consistent with the nature of the target audience. Is the audience English-speaking, are they literate, what is their attitude toward early education and handicapped children? Are they from agencies who view your program as treading on their territory?

It is often necessary to educate the community and parents about the importance of early identification and intervention. Pains must be taken not to alarm or confuse parents unduly, but to provide them with reassurance and a clear explanation of the identification procedures and range of services which will be available.

The public should be provided with the name of a contact person and his telephone number.

WHAT AGENCIES SHOULD BE CONTACTED IN CASEFINDING ACTIVITIES?

Agencies serving both handicapped and nonhandicapped preschool children should be contacted for two reasons: (1) to make them aware of your activities and (2) to enlist their assistance in referring cases to you. Whenever possible, efforts should be made to coordinate and not duplicate services.

Contact with agencies and services might be made through personal interaction or by letter. An exact description of the population to be served as well as the range of services to be provided should be furnished to each agency contacted. Moreover, a contact person and phone number as well as referral form should be provided each agency.

Examples of agencies which should be contacted are: public schools; health services, welfare and social services; community day-care, nursery, and preschool programs; agencies serving handicapped children, such as Easter Seals, United Cerebral Palsy, Crippled Children, Association for Retarded Children; mental health facilities; speech and language clinics; and diagnostic clinics. Private practitioners such as therapists, pediatricians, psychologists, and psychiatrists should also be informed of the availability of program services.

WHAT IS INVOLVED IN A COMMUNITY CANVASS?

One of the most effective casefinding procedures is a door-to-door census which is designed to locate and register all children within a specified age range in the community. This is particularly effective when identifying children with moderate and/or mild impairments or when the objective is to screen all preschool children.

Those doing a door-to-door census may want to conduct a brief parent interview and/or obtain developmental data on the preschool children in the home through questions regarding the mother's prenatal history, child's birth history, the age at which the child walked, talked, etc. In addition, the interviewer may want an opportunity to observe and talk to the child in an informal setting.

The interviewer will also have an opportunity to provide the parents with information on program services, explain the identification procedures, and answer the parents' questions and discuss their concerns. This may be an opportune time to make an appointment for the parents to bring the child in for screening.

Community canvass is an effective technique for registering children, and it may be the only opportunity for talking with parents who have not been reached through other awareness activities. Needless to say, this procedure is time-consuming and may be costly if volunteers are not used. Efforts should be made to develop expedient and inexpensive procedures, in order to avoid detracting funds from the cost of providing services.

Another procedure that is useful in canvassing the community is sending forms home—with school-age children and children in day care, nursery school, and Head Start—on which parents can provide information on preschool children in their families. In addition, a preschool "round-up" can be held during which parents are asked to register their children at designated locations. These two methods are less costly and time-consuming than a door-to-door campaign; they are not as effective, however, in that they rely on parents being literate and cooperative and on the local media being utilized.

WHAT IS THE LAST STEP IN THE CASEFINDING PROCESS?

The last step in the process of locating children is recording referrals and names obtained from the community canvass. Recording procedures should be systematic. Information which needs to be recorded and kept on file is *source of referral, child's name, date of birth, name of parent or guardian*, and *address*, as well as other pertinent information.

WHO SHOULD BE INVOLVED IN THE LOCATION OF CHILDREN FOR SCREENING?

Locating children is a communitywide process. The larger the base of support, the more effective the procedures. All available resources should be contacted and utilized. Examples of resources are:

Newspaper
Radio Stations
Television Stations
Parent Groups (ARCO, ACLD, etc.)

Students From Special Education Departments
Public School Administrators and Teachers
Private School Administrators and Teachers
Pediatricians
Public Health Nurses
Mental Health Staffs
Day-Care and Nursery School Staffs
Head Start Staffs
Caseworkers
Service Organizations (Lions Club, Kiwanis,
  Ladies Aid Society)
League of Women Voters
Clergymen
Developmental Disability Field Workers
Agency Staffs Serving Handicapped Children (Easter Seals,
  UCP, etc.)
Local 4C Members
Municipal Officials

WHO SHOULD COORDINATE THE CASEFINDING PROCESS?

The staff of the agency responsible for casefinding should coordinate the casefinding procedures although all staff should be involved. Often one agency will be responsible for identification and another for providing intervention services for the child. Efforts should be made to establish procedures for coordination and communication between agencies before casefinding and screening begin.

BIBLIOGRAPHY

Hennon, M. L. *Identifying handicapped children for child development programs - A recruitment and selection manual.* Atlanta: Humanics Press, 1974.

Hodskins, D., et al. Guide to recruitment - A manual for head start personnel in recruiting handicapped children. Chapel Hill: Chapel Hill Training - Outreach Project, undated.

Kurtz, D. Child find and screen. An unpublished draft developed as part of the dissemination materials of the HICOMP First Chance Project, Penn State University, University Park, 1975.

Zehrback, R. R. Determining a preschool handicapped population. *Exceptional Children.* 1975, *41*, 76-83.

CHAPTER 3

Screening
David L. Lillie

WHAT IS SCREENING?

Growing up next to a lake, I can remember how we used to catch minnows for fishing bait. Two people would pull a long net with a pole on each end along the bottom of a shallow spot in the lake. The minnows that were only an inch long or smaller would swim through the netting, and we would end up with twenty or thirty, two- to three-inch-long minnows that were just the right size for fishing.

In screening young preschool children, we are essentially going through the same process. Screening is a procedure to separate those children from the population being screened who appear to need special educational services to help them achieve their highest possible functioning level.

WHAT IS THE RELATIONSHIP OF SCREENING TO CASEFINDING AND DIAGNOSIS?

As you become aware of the different measurement activities in the country, it is apparent that *screening* often becomes synonymous with *casefinding* and *diagnosis*. The telescoping of the three activities may be very appropriate in some situations. For example, if the ultimate goal of a state or community is to provide treatment programs for all severely handicapped infants, the following sequence is apt to occur:

DAVID L. LILLIE is Director of the Technical Assistance Development System (TADS) at the University of North Carolina in Chapel Hill. His interests include screening, parent programs, and child development.

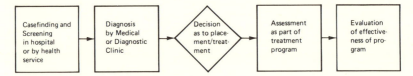

The casefinding and screening processes merge into one activity when it become obvious through the physician or health worker's observation that a child is severely handicapped. As a result of this "eyeball" screening, the infant is referred to a diagnostic center or speciality clinic. Based on the findings from the diagnostic activity, a decision is made concerning treatment.

In the case of mildly handicapped four-year-olds, the differences between the measurement activities are much more distinct. The handicap may not be apparent, which would make "eyeball" casefinding and screening impossible. This fact, plus the age factor, means that the children would probably be at home and would, therefore, have to be "found" or recruited for the screening program. The following sequence of measurement activities would thus be appropriate:

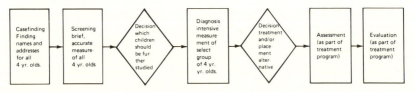

IS SCREENING COSTLY?

Screening becomes an extremely important concept when considering the total amount of time and money available for all the measurement activities from casefinding to evaluation. If screening is conducted *appropriately*, it is a very cost efficient stage in the total helping process, saving the taxpayer a great deal of money and saving the professional a great deal of time. However, if it is confused with diagnosis, especially when considering mildly handicapped populations, screening can be extremely costly in both time and money.

WHAT CAN I FIND OUT ABOUT A CHILD THROUGH SCREENING?

As a result of screening activities, you should have enough information about each child to decide: (1) if he is a candidate for a more thorough diagnostic case study, or (2) if he does not need additional services to maximize his potential (indicating that the prognosis for success without intervention is very good).

WHAT GUIDELINES CAN I FOLLOW TO PLAN A SCREENING PROGRAM?

In the field of medicine, screening for serious conditions and/or diseases has been going on for many years. Recently, medical screening has become more extensive and has indicated screening for various developmental disabilities. Frankenburg and Camp (1975) list ten criteria that should be considered in planning a screening program. In adapting these criteria to planning for educational or developmental screening, six major principles emerge that you should have in mind as decisions are made concerning the screening procedures that will be followed.

1. Screening assumes that the problem being screened for (e.g., developmental delay, emotional maladjustment, or visual impairment) can be ameliorated or modified as a result of subsequent educational treatment programs.

This criterion is familiar to those trained in early childhood or special education. Early intervention studies such as those summarized by Gordon (1968), Caldwell (1970), Lillie (1975), and others offer evidence which indicates that the earlier intervention for handicapped children is provided, the better the results. Other professionals, particularly administrators and decision makers in public schools, are often not so familiar with these studies.

The seriously handicapped preschool child has requirements that make early screening and proper placement especially important. The longer the family alone bears responsibility for the child's welfare, the more likely it is that the family will be debilitated by the burden. Early assistance can modify both the child and the parents' situations.

2. Early intervention (as a result of finding problems early) must improve the condition more than would intervention at a later date when the problem becomes more obvious.

In the case of early education for handicapped children, the exact "best age" of intervention has really not been established. With specific sensory deficits, such as deafness and blindness, we have good empirical evidence that the earlier the intervention, the better. However, with mentally retarded, emotionally disturbed, and learning disabled children, there is no specific evidence indicating that age one intervention is better than age two intervention, or that intervention at age two is better than at age three. What we do have are some general indications, such as those offered by Bloom (1964), that the earlier the intervention, the more there is potential for improvement. This position can certainly be supported by data on the way children develop. Because certain behaviors and skills must be learned before other behaviors and skills can be learned, the untreated child who has difficulty in learning or developing early skills falls further and further behind in his development as time passes.

3. The problem or condition being screened for can be specifically diagnosed through further application of measurement procedures.

Does the child being screened have a handicap that can be specifically diagnosed through additional diagnostic work? This question is more important in medical screening than in educational and developmental screening. In education, screening is the first step in gathering information to make decisions concerning preschool or early childhood intervention. In making such decisions for very young children, the symptoms displayed through behavior—and their "severity"—are more important factors in the total decision-making process than is the physiological cause of the behavior. This is obviously not the case in medicine. If multidisciplinary (education, medicine, etc.) diagnostic personnel and facilities are not available for following through with a determination of placement for a child, however, the time and effort placed into any screening effort should be questioned.

4. The necessary follow-up procedures for next steps are presently or potentially available.

The need for meeting this criterion has been debated. Should you screen and thereby label certain children as handicapped if there are no services available for the children? Uncovering problems without adequate diagnostic treatment facilties does more harm to the child than does not screening for the problem or condition in the first place. We have enough data to demonstrate that when a child is identified as less than adequate, this identification procedure alone will set up reduced expectations on the part of parents, teachers, or any other individual that is aware of the results of that screening activity. When reduced expectations are present, the child's abilities are often shaped to correspond to those expectations.

Presently, the states that have statewide screening programs appear to be assuming that services are potentially available and will be forthcoming. They argue that unless a population of children needing assistance is identified, the necessary funds for providing services will not be allocated.

5. The problem or condition being screened for is relatively prevalent or, the consequences of not discovering a rare problem or condition are very severe.

This criterion is primarily a consideration of the cost in relation to benefit question. Are the potential benefits derived from screening and placement of children worth the cost? If, in other words, you are screening for a relatively rare condition, is the benefit to the few children placed into programs worth the cost? Is the cost worth the results? If the potential number of children that will receive treatment or education are mediocre, the benefits of the program still may be worthwhile because of the number of children involved.

6. Measurement procedures to screen appropriately for the problem should be readily available.

There is a great deal of agreement that measurement procedures are adequate and available. However, there is not substantial agreement among professionals as to what constitutes screening. Most professionals agree that the purpose of screening is ultimately to find those children that need intervention services. However, some screening programs are more diagnostic and/or assessment-oriented (see Chapters 4 and 5) than they are screening-oriented. Thus, the disagreements are not so much over the need for adequate measurement procedures, as much as over the purpose of screening in relation to diagnosis and assessment.

WHO SHOULD CONDUCT SCREENING PROGRAMS?

In many states, the vying for "screening rights" among state agencies is akin to a political football game with no referees in sight. Public health agencies have often taken the lead because of the relationship of developmental screening to physical health screening. The lead agency in screening will vary from state to state or community to community, based on agency capabilities, laws, and political aggressiveness. The important criteria in deciding which agency should coordinate the screening effort are: (1) the screening agency's ability to administer and conduct the screening program efficiently and economically, and (2) its potential for gaining access to follow-up services—such as diagnosis and treatment. Unfortunately, many other factors that have little relevance to these criteria often contribute to the decisions.

WHAT GROUP OF INDIVIDUALS WILL CONDUCT THE SCREENING SESSIONS?

Past practices have indicated that paraprofessionals or nondegree child workers can be trained to administer standardized screening instruments efficiently and objectively. Some programs use volunteers, such as members of the Junior Service League. Often, the administrative problem of utilizing individuals whose time is not controlled by a salary reinforcement is not worth the funds that a volunteer program might save you.

WHICH AGE GROUP OF PRESCHOOL CHILDREN SHOULD BE SCREENED FIRST?

Because intervention should be started as soon as problems are detected (and the earlier, the better), screening would logically, it seems, be done first with infants. It has been argued convincingly, however, that service—once begun—should be continuous, without gaps. To make sure that infants will receive continuous service as they pass through the preschool years, it is necessary to have programs for ages one to five before programs for infants. In other words, if you want a program without gaps in continuous service, screening should be begun with the oldest children first. Currently, some states are beginning with the younger children while others are starting to screen the older children first.

CAN'T YOU PLACE CHILDREN DIRECTLY INTO PROGRAMS AS SOON AS THEY ARE SCREENED?

Even though programs can be found that do place children into treatment activities as a result of screening procedures, they are taking a chance that many children will be inappropriately placed and treated. Again, using screening in this way is not as serious when, at screening, the problems of the child are quite obvious and severe. Generally, however, a measurement activity that provides enough information to enable you to make a placement decision is much more than screening; it is diagnosis.

WHAT KINDS OF MEASUREMENT INSTRUMENTS SHOULD BE USED FOR SCREENING?

There are several criteria to consider. First, instruments used must be standardized. The major pupose of screening—to sort out those children from the general population who need further study— dictates the use of measurement devices that compare that child with the general population. Therefore, the procedures used for the development of the test must meet acceptable standards for the collection of normative data. In addition, the tests and measurement procedures must be administered in a standardized manner to assure accurate comparison to the general population. Second, the screening test should be easily, quickly, and economically administered. Third, the test or measurement should accurately sort out the children who need further study with as few mistakes as possible. Fourth, the test should be acceptable to the professionals who are going to do the follow-up work, both at the diagnostic level and at the treatment or educational level, as well as to parents and the general public.

The chart on the following page, which presents several tests that meet most of these criteria, is not an all-inclusive list of acceptable screening instruments, but it is representative of those being used across the country today. In my estimation, a number of the screening instruments available meet the necessary selection criteria, and there is no need to go to the expense and time of developing your own instrument to reflect the uniqueness of your community or state. Certainly, there is always a professional need to seek and develop better instruments. This activity should be considered, however, for what it is—a research and development effort, the end results of which may lead to effective use of the new instrument. If the main goal of your effort is screening, as defined here, you will serve yourself and the taxpayer more appropriately by selecting an instrument already developed and proven effective.

CHARACTERISTICS OF SEVERAL SELECTED PRESCHOOL SCREENING TESTS

TEST	AGE RANGE	INDIVIDUAL OR GROUP	TIME TO ADMINISTER	WHO ADMINISTERS	STANDARDIZATION	VALIDITY	RELIABILITY
DENVER DEVELOPMENTAL SCREENING TEST	0-6	Individual	15-25 min	designed for people who have not had training in psychological testing	Standardized 1,036 blue and white collar children	High agreement between DDST and quotients of Stanford Binet and Bayley	95.8% test-retest reliability 90% among examiners
ALPERN-BOLL	0-11	Individual	20-40 min	teacher or nurse	Standardized on 3008 subjects	Validity in determining developmental ages of black and white urban mid-Americans of all social classes. Validity index of 86% of mother's report of skills as compared to test academic scales demonstrate validity to standard I.Q. tests.	Extremely high scorer and test retest reliability
DIAL	2½-5½	Individual	20-30 min	team administered - trained paraprofessional	Normed on 40,000 children	RESEARCH OVER 3 YEARS FOR PREDICTIVE RELIABILITY AND VALIDITY.	
ABC INVENTORY	3.9-4.11	Individual	20 min	teacher	Sampled on 480 children. Scores were not separated according to sex nor was SES considered.	78 correlation between ABC and Stanford Binet. Predictive validity based on first grade pass fail	Reliability based on high similarity from measures of location and dispersion for sample group

BIBLIOGRAPHY

Bloom, B. *Stability and change in human characteristics*. New York: John Wiley, 1964.

Caldwell, B. *Preschool inventory* (rev. ed.). Princeton: Educational Testing Service, 1970

Gordon, T. *Studying the child in schools.* New York: John Wiley, 1966.

Lillie, D. *Early childhood education: An individualized approach to developmental instruction*. Chicago: Science Research Associates, 1975.

CHAPTER 4

Diagnosis
Art Cross

WHAT IS DIAGNOSIS?

Diagnosis is a process designed: (1) to confirm or disconfirm the existence of a problem, serious enough to require remediation, in those children identified in a screening effort and (2) to clarify the nature of the problem (is it organic, environmental, or both?). The primary purpose of diagnosis is to provide enough information about a child's condition to allow an intelligent decision to be made on the appropriate placement of the child into a treatment program.

HOW DOES DIAGNOSIS DIFFER FROM SCREENING AND ASSESSMENT?

Screening "samples" a child's abilities in various areas while diagnosis involves an in-depth examination of problems uncovered during screening. Also, screening can often be done by paraprofessionals, while diagnosis must involve professionals from a variety of fields such as medicine (to provide information on physiological problems), psychology (to provide information on behavioral problems), and education (to help in deciding on the best instructional route for the child).

Assessment is concerned primarily with the development of specific educational (remediation) procedures while diagnosis is concerned with finding an appropriate medical or educational program in which to place the child. In other words, diagnosis iden-

ART CROSS, formerly an Assistant Professor of Special Education at Chicago State University, is pursuing a doctoral degree at the University of North Carolina in Chapel Hill. His interests include teacher training, program development for young children, and parent training.

25

tifies the *kind* of treatment while assessment determines the *content* of the treatment.

CAN YOU GIVE EXAMPLES ILLUSTRATING THE RELATIONSHIPS BETWEEN DIAGNOSIS AND SCREENING AND ASSESSMENT?

Yes. If a *screening* test showed that a child had a sore throat, *diagnostic* tests would be run to determine the cause of the problem (bacteria, virus, etc.) which would help the diagnosticians determine the appropriate kind of treatment (no treatment, antibiotic treatment, treatment of symptoms such as fever). An *assessment* procedure would be used to determine the content of the treatment—the specific drugs or other therapy.

Similarly, a child who scored low on expressive language ability in a *screening* examination would have to be *diagnosed* to determine the exact causes for his poor performance. These causes could range from retardation or lack of emphasis on speaking at home to a lack of motivation to speak for the screening examiners. Each of the possible causes would probably be best remediated by a particular intervention approach (e.g., a home-based program, a center-based program, etc.). The personnel at the program selected would conduct an *assessment* of the child to determine the *content* of his individual program.

HOW SHOULD THE DIAGNOSTIC PROCESS BEGIN?

It should begin with the diagnosticians asking two questions: (1) What type of data do I need on this child? and (2) What kinds and amounts of data can I consider sufficient evidence of ability or disability in the suspect area(s)? The answer to the first question will help in making decisions on the types of personnel and equipment that will be needed to gather data. The answer to the second question, of course, will be used to pinpoint problems.

WHAT PROCESSES ARE INVOLVED IN DIAGNOSIS?

A number, the most important of which are ANALYSIS—which involves collecting data on various areas of concern with the child—and SYNTHESIS—which involves examining the results of the analysis and developing a comprehensive interpretation of the results.

ANALYSIS

What are typical areas of investigation in the analysis phase?
Those listed in TABLE 1 are typical. It may be unnecessary to investigate all of the areas listed because of the information already available from the screening test. This information (on the major need or delay area, such as language, motor, cognitive, or social) should guide the prescription of tests. The following sequence of events is useful in diagnostic examination:

    1. Diagnose physical functioning first (medical and other health-related areas) to rule out or detect specific organic impairments (Kaufmann and Hallahan, 1974).

    2. Second, obtain an accurate, in-depth history of the child which details pertinent antecedent data (Brown, 1973).

    3. Observation of the child should come last.[1] It should focus on at least three areas: (a) parent-child interaction; (b) child-object interaction; (c) child-other interaction.

What personnel are involved? The need for personnel should be determined by the type of diagnosis required. Some of the possible personnel would be: social worker, pediatrician, neurologist, psychologist, public health nurse, and educational specialist. Do not involve people unnecessarily in data collection unless their expertise is genuinely warranted. For example, do not request psychiatric services for *mild* emotional problems. Do not ask other specialists to continue diagnosing a *child* if all the information you have suggests the problem area has been found.

Parents should also be involved in the diagnostic process. They have a *right* to be involved in the following ways:

    1. in information-giving and data collection;

    2. in reacting to the information accumulated (e.g., how similar is the sampled behavior to the child's "usual" behavior?);

    3. as full participants in the decision-making process surrounding consideration of placement/treatment alternatives;

    4. as recipients of the best information available concerning the status of their child and what they may expect in the future.

What tools should be used in analysis? There is no one individual diagnostic test. A battery of diagnostic tools which is capable of

---

[1]Simeonsson and Wiegerink (1975) emphasize the need for the "behavior of the child (to) be systematically observed in his environmental context to determine the functional relationship which antecedent or consequent events may have on his behavior" (p. 477).

TABLE 1

TYPICAL AREAS OF INVESTIGATION IN DIAGNOSIS

Area of Investigation	Personnel Involved	Type of Information Obtained
(1) Social History	Social Worker	Information relative to the functioning of the total family unit; note what the child's problem means to the family.
(2) Physical Examination	Pediatrician	Child's general health at present; review the child's medical history; note any physical defects that may be present.
(3) Neurological Examination	Neurologist	Specific information of any central nervous system impairment if brain damage is suspected; run an EEG to detect possibility of seizures or other malfunctioning.
(4) Psychological Examination	Psychologist	Data from the administration of psychometric techniques; use diagnostic tests to measure child's performance against normative standards and projective tests to determine nature of child's emotional responses.
(5) Hearing Examination	Audiologist or Public Health Worker	Data from the application of audiometric procedures to determine any type of hearing impairment.
(6) Vision Examination	Opthamologist or Public Health Worker	Detection of any visual impairment.
(7) Speech Examination	Speech Pathologist	Child's ability to understand and/or use words, phrases, concepts.
(8) Educational Examination	Special Education/ Early Childhood	Diagnostic instruction to determine child's learning style and abilities (general here; more specific within the area of Assessment).

yielding a picture of the child which reflects the complexity of the human condition should be applied. Such a battery includes at least four types of data collection: interview, history, observation, and standardized instruments.

1. Interview—These may be structured or unstructured. The former tend to garner specific information more quickly than the latter, although a wealth of informative data can be gained from unstructured (digressive) interviews. Essentially, the interview should be designed to obtain a detailed description of the current behavior of the child. Palmer (1970) suggests this description should include "the ways in which the parents have attempted to deal with the child's behavior, and their feelings and attitudes about it" (p. 119). Also see Hauessermann, 1958.

2. History—All pertinent antecedent data, or at least considerable detail about the child's past development and the situations affecting it, should be noted here. Palmer (1970) states that such a history is vital "since it provides an estimate of both the rate of development and some of the past stresses or continuous stresses that may affect the child's current status" (p. 119). The major technique used for preparing a history is a bibliographical data sheet. In Figure 1 (adapted from Brown, 1973), areas one may consider in preparing a history are displayed.

3. Observation—Certain guidelines should be followed when reporting and drawing inferences concerning children's behavior. The two major ones are: (a) define how and where the child was observed, and (b) specify the length and frequency of observation. Observations are valuable in detecting patterns or themes in the child's behavior as well as in noting reactions that may be limited to a specific kind of situation. Observations may be made in structured as well as unstructured settings. One may wish to describe all that occurs or look only for certain designated behaviors. A recording system which allows accurate analysis of the data obtained via observation is necessary.

4. Standardized Instruments—The past decade has seen an increasingly larger number of available standardized instruments; the existence of numerous excellent reviews (Gallagher, 1972; TADS, 1972; and CSE/ECRC, 1971) makes their discussion here unnecessary. In a review, Gallagher (1972) questions the technical adequacy of many of these instruments. His remarks hopefully will provide our readers with some guidance in the crucial area of test selection:

> The rapidly growing number of 'tests' designed to measure all types of psychological functions and the great demand from a relatively unsophisticated

FIGURE 1

AREAS OFTEN COVERED ON
GENERAL CASE HISTORY FORMS

1. **BIRTH HISTORY**

   Previous pregnancies
   Miscarriages
   Mother's health/attitude
   Labor
   Delivery
   Birth Weight
   Trouble breathing, sucking
   Jaundice, cyanosis
   Oxygen

2. **MOTOR DEVELOPMENT**

   Sat alone
   Crawled
   Fine and gross motor coordi-
     nation
   Feeding, sucking, chewing
   Drooling
   Toilet training
   Enuresis
   Self-help

3. **LANGUAGE**

   Comprehension
   Gestures
   Echolalia
   Perserveration
   Onset of words
   Current number of words
   Onset of sentences
   Examples of sentences
   % understood by parents
   % understood by other adults
   % understood by siblings
   % understood by peers
   Child's awareness of problem
   Previous assessment
   Previous training

4. **FAMILY**

   Parent's age, health
   Parent's occupation
   Parent's education
   Parent's income
   Marital status
   Is child adopted
   Siblings; age, health
   Others in home; age, health
   History of learning problems in
     family

(4. **FAMILY, Con't.**)

   Other problems
   Language spoken in home
   Transportation

5. **INTERPERSONAL RELATION-
   SHIPS**

   General disposition
   Playmates and play habits
   Parent-child relationships
   Other adult relationships
   In contact with environment
   Discipline
   Affectionate
   Aggressive
   Compulsive
   Cries easily
   Daydreamer
   Fears
   Hyperactive
   Jealousy
   Leader or follower
   Perservation
   Sleep habits
   Social perception
   Tantrums
   Psychological assessment(s)
   Psychological treatment(s)
   Psychiatric assessment(s)
   Psychiatric treatment(s)

6. **MEDICAL HISTORY**

   Convulsions
   Fever
   Childhood diseases
   Cerebral problem(s)
   Glandular disturbance
   Excessive sweating
   Allergies
   Drug therapy
   Auditory problems
   Vision problems
   Operation
   Accidents
   Congenital defects
   Name of doctor

7. **ADDITIONAL COMMENTS**

set of users for these tests underscore the responsibility of the professions to see to it that the Standards for Educational and Psychological Tests, jointly established oy the American Psychological Association and the American Educational Research Association (25), are observed.

Below are listed only a few of these standards which the reader is encouraged to match against the latest release of a new test of perception or of language development or whatever for preschool children.

A2 The test and its manual should be revised at appropriate intervals. While no universal rule can be given, it would appear proper in most circumstances for the publisher to withdraw a test from the market if the manual is fifteen or more years old and no revision can be obtained.

B2 The test manual should state implicitly the purposes and applications for which the test is recommended.

B3 The test manual should indicate the qualifications required to administer the test and to interpret it properly.

C1 The manual should report the validity of the test for each type of inference for which it is recommended.

C5 The sample employed in a validity study and the conditions under which testing is done should be consistent with the recommendations made in the manual.

F5 Norms should be reported in the test manual in terms of standard scores or percentile ranks which reflect the distribution of scores in an appropriate reference group or groups (Gallagher, 1972, p. 104).

SYNTHESIS

What do you mean by "synthesis?" Bringing together the results of all the analyses so that they form an accurate picture of the child's condition is called synthesis. Generally, the diagnostic team and the parents are involved in the synthesis process. This is because each result must be evaluated carefully in light of all the other results—by people with expertise in the various areas and by people who know the child intimately—to prevent misinterpretation of the meaning of the results in terms of the total child.

What is involved in synthesis? First, all data must be considered. Then, patterns in the child's behavior, abilities, etc., as revealed by the data, must be ascertained. Finally, the meaning of the findings must be explored in order to place the child in a program; this is done in what is called an interpretive or case conference.

Such a conference involves a meeting of all persons who have pertinent diagnostic information or are involved in the placement decision. Due process regulations require the presence of parents. If parents are excluded from this meeting, a separate conference must be held to inform them of the finding of the first conference. This latter arrangement can cause confusion and mistrust.

What happens during an interpretive conference? The following is a suggested sequence of a desirable procedure. First, all participants must be made aware of the procedures to be used in the conference. Then, the significant findings of each participant should be considered. Next, consensus must be reached on a "profile" of the child's major needs. Then, the placement options should be reviewed, the constraints and resources of each option in terms of the child should be determined, and a decision on placement which is based on the best match with the needs of the child and family should be made. Finally, responsibilities should be designated: i.e., what agency is held responsible for service, what are the responsibilities of the parents, and who is to be responsible for the transfer of records?

HOW MUCH DIAGNOSIS SHOULD THERE BE?

When the diagnostic team agrees on the child's needs and the appropriate placement, there has been enough diagnosis to make some decisions about treatment. Certainly, a child should be "treated" as soon as it is reasonably clear that a particular treatment is indicated.

WHAT ABOUT KEEPING RECORDS?

The information gained throughout the diagnostic process must be stored in a useful manner. Utility may be considered in terms of accessibility, understandability, and usefulness. These three criteria necessitate a systematic record-keeping procedure. The reason for keeping records is because of their usefulness to the personnel who facilitate the educational assessment/treatment/assessment cycle. The ultimate goal of the diagnostic process is informed decision making. Specifically, the process attempts to make it possible to answer two questions: "What is inhibiting the child's development?" and "What will best facilitate his optimal development?"

WHAT ARE THE SOURCES OF ERROR IN DEVELOPMENTAL DIAGNOSIS?

Many are possible. Table 2 suggests a few of our present limitations in diagnosis.

TABLE 2

SOURCES OF ERROR IN DEVELOPMENTAL DIAGNOSIS

Source	Possible Errors
(1) History	Failure to take a thorough history; undue reliance on the past without allowing for possibility of change.
(2) Interpretation	Incorrect assumption of inability caused by child's failure to co-operate; failure to note the quality of the child's performance; failure to withhold judgment in case of doubt.
(3) Observation	Limited setting (i.e., diagnostic center only as opposed to combination of multiple settings); single observations rather than observations of greater duration and frequency; decontextualization of the testing situation.
(4) Instrumentation	Lack of multiple measures; administration by unskilled personnel; overemphasis on "objective" data.
(5) Placement	Lack of available options; no consideration of existing options.

BIBLIOGRAPHY

Brown, Diana. *Developmental handicaps in babies and young children.* Springfield, Ill.: Charles C. Thomas, 1973.

Gallagher, James and Bradley, Robert. Early identification of developmental difficulties. *Yearbook of the National Society for the Study of Education, Part II (vol. 71).* Chicago: University of Chicago Press, 1972.

Gorham, Kathryn; Des Jardin, Charlotte; Page, Ruth; Pettis, Eugene; and Sheilber, Barbara. Effect on parents. In Nicholas Hobbs (ed.), *Issues in the classification of children* (vol. I). San Francisco: Jossey-Bass, 1975.

Grim, J. (ed.). *Evaluation bibliography.* Chapel Hill: TADS, 1973.

Hauessermann, Else. *Developmental potential of preschool children.* New York: Grune and Stratton, 1958.

Hoepfner, Ralph; Stern, Carolyn; and Nummedal, Ed. *CSE/ECRC preschool kindergarten test evaluations.* Los Angeles: UCLA Graduate School of Education, 1971.

Kaufmann, James and Hallahan, Daniel. The medical model and the science of special education. *Exceptional Children,* 1974, *41,* 97-101.

Lickorish, J.R. The psychometric assessment of the family. In John Howells (ed.), *Theory and practice of family psychiatry.* New York: Brunner, Mazel, 1971.

Palmer, James. *The psychological assessment of children.* New York: John Wiley & Sons, Inc., 1970.

Simeonsson, Rune and Wiegerink, Ronald. Accountability: A dilemma in infant intervention. *Exceptional Children,* 1975, *41,* 474-481.

CHAPTER 5

Educational Assessment
Gloria Harbin

WHAT IS ASSESSMENT?

Assessment is the systematic process of (1) *collecting* information both on a child's level of functioning in specific areas of development and on his learning characteristics and (2) carefully *interpreting* the information which is collected. The purpose of assessment is to develop a comprehensive and specific educational plan which provides the information that is necessary in planning a day-to-day program for the child. Unlike diagnosis, which allows general areas in which a child is having difficulty to be defined, assessment attempts to determine specific strengths and weaknesses in the child's abilities, as well as his level of functioning and learning characteristics. For example, diagnosis may reveal that a child is functioning at a three-year-old level in developing motor skills and is especially having difficulty in developing gross motor or large muscle skills. Assessment will reveal the specific problem skills: such as balancing on one foot, walking up stairs with alternating feet, and hesitancy to attempt or participate in activities that require gross motor skills.

WHAT SKILLS NEED TO BE ASSESSED?

Those in the following developmental areas:
1. Gross motor or large muscle development (running, sitting, and throwing);

GLORIA HARBIN, formerly an Early Childhood Program Specialist at the Mid-East Learning Resource System in Chapel Hill, is pursuing a doctoral degree at the University of North Carolina. Her interests include assessment, curriculum, and teacher training.

2. Fine motor or small muscle development (grasping, bead stringing, cutting, and writing);
3. Visual perceptual (visual discrimination between likenesses and differences, visual closure, figure-ground, and spatial relationships);
4. Reasoning (associations, classification, part-whole relationships, sequencing, and quantitative skills);
5. Receptive language (the meaningful interpretation of what is seen and heard, such as following one step commands);
6. Expressive language (the gestures and speech that communicate wants or ideas to others, such as the use of simple sentences and the use of regular plurals); and
7. Social and emotional (the child's feelings about himself and his interactions with adults, peers, and the environment).

Because the developmental areas are interrelated, it is impossible to separate skills in one area totally from skills in another. In assessment, however, it is imperative that the child's strengths and weaknesses be specified clearly. Exact delineation of skill areas during the assessment helps in finding specific problems. If "fine motor" and "perception" are grouped together, for example, it is often difficult to tell whether the child is experiencing difficulty in the development of fine motor skills, whether he is unable to do the task because of faulty perceptual development or whether the problem is intersensory integration.

It is important to assess the child's ability to adapt to his home and community environment (adaptive behavior). The assessment of adaptive behavior (in terms of the seven developmental areas) allows more insight into the child's functioning level than an assessment which concerns only the child's abilities within the educational setting. The latter type of assessment sometimes results in a very narrow, biased view of the child.

WHAT GUIDELINES CAN I FOLLOW IN COLLECTING AND INTERPRETING ASSESSMENT INFORMATION?

There are several:

1. *Assessment of the child should be systematic, thorough, and accurate.* Many people collect information in a haphazard manner which leaves gaps that make interpretation of the data unreliable or inappropriate. Some people collect information relatively well, but they do not interpret the results carefully and systematically. The purpose of assessment is not to label the child but to collect and interpret (carefully) enough information to develop a specific educational plan. The degree to which assessment is systematic,

thorough, and accurate determines the degree to which the educational plan is relevant and effective.

2. *The teacher should conduct the assessment using input from the parents and other professionals.* Parents are often able to give pertinent information concerning the skills and behaviors that the child uses outside the classroom.

The teacher is the best and most logical person to assess the child's skills for a number of reasons. First, he* can capitalize on both the child's familiarity with the surroundings and the rapport that's developed during the educational process. These factors help in obtaining an accurate view of the child's abilities. Second, when the teacher assesses the child, he observes the learning style or characteristics of the child. This knowledge will be helpful later in the teaching situation. Third, the teacher is the person who most urgently needs the assessment information in order to develop an individual plan for the child. Results from diagnosis are often slow in coming to the teacher, and once they arrive they are often too general to help with specific day-to-day programming.

3. *Assessment should be a part of an ongoing instructional process.* Assessment is not a one-time occurrence. After the child has been assessed, an educational plan is written. The teacher then begins teaching the child skills and assessing his progress. In other words, assessment occurs over and over again throughout the year.

4. *Assessment should be conducted after the child becomes used to the teacher or the home-trainer and the classroom setting.* If information is not collected in accordance with this guideline then the interpretations are suspect and may be inaccurate.

5. *It is important to assess the child using his native language.* Unless the child's native language is used, it is impossible to determine what and how much the child actually knows or can do. For example, if a child is bilingual and does not respond to a request given in standard English, we cannot be sure whether the child was unable to respond because (a) he did not have the skill or, (b) he did not understand the request.

It is also important in the area of language to ascertain which standard English language structures and content the child is able to understand (receptive) and use (expressive). Since standard English is the primary language in this country, it is important to increase the child's skills in this area so that he will not be denied mobility.

6. *When the child has a known handicap (such as cerebral palsy, a hearing impairment, or a visual impairment) the nature of the*

*Masculine pronoun is used generically. As often as not, the teacher is female.

handicap should be kept in mind during the collection and interpretation of the assessment information. Sometimes it might be necessary to make adjustments in an item because of the child's handicapping condition. Consequently, it is extremely important to determine the actual skill that an item or task is designed to assess. Consider, for example, the following: "Is able to copy three designs." The item appears in the "visual perception" section of the assessment device. The ability to draw the designs, however, is only a "vehicle" for assessing how well the child perceives the designs. If the child being assessed has a motor impairment, the design could be made with large styrofoam strips and the child could be allowed to copy the design using the styrofoam. Unfortunately, it is not always possible to alter a task in light of a child's handicapping condition. Further information concerning techniques for adapting items for certain handicapping conditions can be found in Haeusserman (1958).

7. *The child's prior experiences influence his concepts and his abilities.* Children from different geographical areas, socioeconomic backgrounds, ethnic groups, and residences (urban-rural) often have widely differing experiences. In collecting and interpreting assessment information, all children should not be assumed to have similar backgrounds. For a child growing up in the country (rural area), for example, there is a difference between a picture which depicts "night-time" in the city (urban area) and one which depicts "night-time" in the country. If the child does not recognize a picture of night-time in the city as "night-time," it is unclear whether the child: (a) does not know the concept of "night-time" or (b) does not know the concept of "night-time in the city." It is, of course, important to assess the child across cultural, regional, and ethnic concepts in order to determine: (a) how much he knows about his environment and, (b) what things he does not know but perhaps needs to know to be more mobile.

8. *Some combination of norm-referenced, criterion-referenced, observation, and Piagetian devices should be used for assessment.* The use of only one type of device cannot give the teacher the broadest possible picture of the child. Interpretations of the child's performance based only upon observation or only upon norm-referenced devices usually do not result in an accurate picture of the child's functioning level.

9. *The instruments and procedures used to collect information should give as much accurate and pertinent information as possible.* There are many norm-referenced and criterion-referenced tests available today. Some are very good while others are inadequate for use either with preschool handicapped children as a

group or for a particular type of handicapped child. Several devices and observation procedures should be examined to ascertain which ones are the most appropriate for assessing the children in each educational setting. The instruments and procedures used should yield valid information and not penalize the children because of culture or sex. In cases where the information is biased in favor of white middle-class culture, the teacher must use systematic observation techniques and criterion-referenced devices which are based upon developmental milestones, to balance the bias and obtain an accurate picture of the child's strengths and weaknesses.

10. *During the assessment, a number of variables may affect the child's performance and thus influence the manner in which data should be collected*. The following is only a partial list of the possible variables. The teacher should keep these in mind in order to insure the child's best performance during the assessment.

    a. Position — The position of the materials might make it easier or harder for a child to choose the correct response.

    b. Size of materials — If the materials are too large or too small, the child will have a difficult time handling or seeing them.

    c. Color of materials — For some children, color is distracting.

    d. Length of the session — If the session is too long, the child will become fatigued. It is then likely that he will refuse to do tasks or will do them poorly.

    e. Attending skills — Some children are labeled as "untestable" because they have poor attending skills. Attending skills are crucial for the child to be able to focus on, understand, and perform a task.

    f. Attention span — Attention span varies among children. If a child has a short attention span, sessions should be shorter.

    g. Reinforcement — For some children, it is extremely important to reinforce not the answers but the responding behavior. The child must be encouraged to feel positive about the situation.

    h. Distractions — Materials on the table, a cluttered room, and noise are just a few of the possible distractions that might affect the child's performance.

    i. Time of day — During some periods of the day, children are more fatigued and distractible.

    j. Comfort and accessibility of materials — Is the child sitting in a chair that is appropriate to his size? If not, it might alter fine motor and visual perceptual skills enough for the child to be unable to respond correctly.

    k. Initial success or failure — This will set the tone and determine whether a child will continue to respond and give his best performance.

l. Telling rather than asking — Tell the child in a kind and gentle but firm manner, "Make one like this." If you say, "Will you" or "Do you want to," he may respond by saying "No."

m. Order of assessment — It is best to begin an assessment with activities that do not upset a child to the point that other activities cannot be performed. For example, assessing gross motor skills tends to raise the activity level of the child. The increase in activity level may reduce the ability of an easily distracted child to attend to the subsequent task. Similarly, activities that require high energy or interaction with people might frighten a child.

n. Modeling or demonstration — Some tasks are not supposed to be demonstrated. For those tasks that require demonstration, the teacher should be aware that the manner in which he demonstrates will affect the child's response.

HOW SHOULD DATA OR INFORMATION BE COLLECTED?

A combination of criterion-referenced devices, norm-referenced devices, Piagetian devices, and observation techniques is generally the best way of obtaining the information on a child's level of development that is needed to develop an educational program. The most important guides to the proper use of these approaches are the individual child and the teacher's judgment. Rarely can all the information needed about a child for developing a program be obtained from instruments alone or observations alone. A teacher must tailor the approach he uses for assessment to each child. The data he cannot obtain by using criterion-referenced tools must be obtained through observation, or norm-referenced devices, and vice versa.

HOW CAN NORM-REFERENCED DEVICES BE USED?

The purpose of a norm-referenced measure is to show how the child's performance compares to the performance of other children who are the same chronological age. Norm-referenced devices must be valid and reliable. Some norm-referenced devices are able to give the teacher in-depth information in one area of development, such as language. There are those who feel the Illinois Test of Psycholinguistic Abililities (ITPA) or the Developmental

Sentence Analysis, for example, provide in-depth information on the language abilities of young children.

Many norm-referenced devices have a limited number of items which are not in developmental sequences. Thus, the information obtained from such devices is often general, and only confirms suspicions that the child is functioning below others who are the same chronological age. This limitation is especially true in the case of intelligence tests.

HOW CAN CRITERION-REFERENCED DEVICES BE USED?

The purpose of a criterion-referenced device is to compare the child not to other children but to a set of standards. This set of standards is usually developed by selecting items from several standardized (norm-referenced) developmental tests, such as the "Bayley Scales of Infant Development" or the "Developmental Diagnosis" by Arnold Gesell. Criterion-referenced devices developed in this manner usually cover most of the developmental areas listed earlier in this chapter and contain items listed in developmental sequence within each developmental area. This allows the teacher to determine the level at which the child is functioning and to measure the child's progress from one point in time to another, not in terms of an overall score (as with norm-referenced devices) but in terms of specific developmental skills. The purpose of developmental, criterion-referenced devices is concisely described by Sanford.when she states, "The teacher is not absorbed with the child's chronological age, intellectual level, or comparisons with other youngsters, but is concerned with focusing on the next specific appropriate skill to be taught to the particular child" (Sanford, 1975). Hence, criterion-referenced devices are designed to facilitate daily programming for children.

The recent surge in the development and use of criterion-referenced devices with preschool handicapped children has raised three major questions among early education professionals, such as educators, psychologists, and administrators. First, should a criterion-referenced device be valid and reliable? Most professionals agree that criterion-referenced tests should be reliable and valid, but not in the same way as norm-referenced devices (Cox, 1973; Carver, 1973). In criterion-referenced tools, reliability and validity are linked to the ability of the device to show differences (growth or progress) within an individual rather than between individuals. Content validity is immensely important because the content of the criterion-referenced assessment device becomes the basis of the child's educational program.

Secondly, the question of whether or not it is appropriate to use a norm-referenced test in a criterion-referenced manner arises. Most agree it is appropriate only after careful scrutiny of the device. It is important to determine whether the criteria (items on the norm-referenced device) are compatible with the goals and objectives of your program. Some devices lend themselves more to this use than do others. The "Preschool Inventory" is an example of a norm-referenced device that has been used widely in a criterion-referenced manner. On the other hand, intelligence tests do not lend themselves as easily to use as a criterion-referenced measure.

Third, who is qualified to develop a criterion-referenced device? Many people have developed these devices. It is not something that is done only by researchers, psychologists, psychometrians, and professional test developers. In fact, many teachers have been involved in developing criterion-referenced measures (Bangs, 1975). Because of the number of the devices and the range of individuals developing them, however, the quality is varied. If you are interested in developing your own criterion-referenced assessment tool, it might be helpful to review other devices first. If one of the other assessment tools meets the needs of your program (or with some adaption meets the needs), it would save you from "reinventing the wheel." The bibliography at the end of this publication lists several criterion-referenced assessment devices. (See Figure 1.)

WHAT ARE THE STRENGTHS AND WEAKNESSES OF CRITERION-REFERENCED TOOLS?

Strengths: (1) They are concerned with measuring the individual growth and progress of the child instead of comparing him to others of his own chronological age. They are, thus, a way of recording and measuring the progress of each child. (2) Criterion-referenced devices are usually sequenced developmentally, allowing teachers to know exactly which skill or skills to work on next. In other words, the devices assist teachers in writing specific instructional objectives for each child. (3) They usually cover many developmental areas, whereas normative devices often cover only one area of development. (4) They usually have more items than norm-referenced devices, and thereby provide smaller steps for measuring each developmental area. (5) They allow flexibility in administration and new items can be developed when necessary. Their major goal is to determine whether a child can do a particular

Figure 1

SAMPLE PAGE
FROM CRITERION
REFERENCED TEST

VISUAL PERCEPTION

Task Number	Description	D.A.*	Can Do	Cannot Do
1	*Matches color to sample.* Present child with six different color cubes. Keep a matching set of six out of sight, presenting them one at a time and asking him to show you one just like it. Do not name the color, or ask child to do so. Demonstrate. Five correct for pass.	2	___	___
2	*Groups things together by color, form, or size.* Examples: colored blocks, poker chips, or marbles; different size blocks, cups, or logs, different forms such as shapes, beads, or silverware (knives, forks, spoons). Does this during play.	2	___	___
3	*Stacks five rings on a peg in order.* Demonstrate. Rings should be of graduated sizes. Pass if the child is able to give you the rings in the correct order but has trouble stacking them on the peg. The objective of this item is to see whether the child can perceive (visually) differences in size—not the fine-motor ability to stack.	2	___	___
4	*Matches to sample circle, square, and triangle.* Present child with templates (two each) for the above shapes. Picks up circle, asking child to find another like it. Return circle templates to the group. Repeat for square and triangle. Allow one trial for each shape. Three correct for pass.	3	___	___
5	*Makes circle out of two half circles after demonstration.* Present halves to child with edges parellel to edge of table in front of child. Allow three trials.	3	___	___
6	*Matches to sample pictures of animals: dog, horse, bear, and cat.* Point to one of the pictures in the top row and ask child to "find one like this one." Repeat for the three other pictures. Must get all correct.	3	___	___
7	*Name pictures of items removed from view.* Show child three culturally familiar pictures and name them. Hide pictures from view one at a time until each has been hidden once. Three correct for pass.	4	___	___
8	*Selects two identical pictures out of set of three.* Ask child to point to the two pictures that are exactly alike. Three correct for pass.	4	___	___
9	*Adds two parts to an incomplete man.* Tell child to draw in the parts that are missing. Pass anything that resembles an arm and leg. See page 14	4	___	___
10	*Copies three designs.* Allow two trials for each design. Ask child to "make one just like this one." Draw each of the following designs one at a time for the child. He must copy the design using crayon or primary pencil. The objective of this item is to see if the child can visually perceive these designs not if he has fine-motor ability to draw. Pass any design that perceptually resembles the one you drew.	5	___	___
11	*Put together a large four-to six-piece puzzle after demonstration.*	5	___	___
12	*Arranges coins from smallest to largest (dime, nickle, quarter, half dollar).* Demonstrate and describe task. Allow two trials. One correct for pass.	5	___	___

*Developmental Age

Developmental Age Ceiling (highest age level at which child can do two or more tasks): _____

Task that child cannot do *at and below* Developmental Age Ceiling: _____

Long-Range Objectives (by task number): _____

Notes and Comments: _____

_____
_____

*Reprinted from *The Carolina Developmental Profile* (D. Lillie and G. Harbin). Winston-Salem: Kaplan School Supply, 1976.

task. (6) The person who most needs information for programming is the person who uses the criterion-referenced device.

Weaknesses: (1) Many criterion-referenced devices are designed for use with certain groups of children. In trying to use the device with a group of children other than those intended, the teacher may discover that the device is inappropriate or of little value because it does not measure skills of concern with his children. (2) Criterion-referenced devices are often specific. Consequently, they tend to measure what some people call "splinter skills." They concentrate on parts of a larger skill area. The use of a criterion-referenced assessment device, therefore, does not yield a total picture of the child. (3) Children go through two stages in developing skills: acquisition and generalization. Criterion-referenced devices tend to measure only acquisition. For example, a child who is able to hold his spoon and eat food of a particular texture in one setting has acquired a skill; when he is able to use his spoon in other settings and eat foods of various textures, his skill has become generalized. The item on the criterion-referenced assessment device, "Is able to use spoon," depends for an accurate assessment on the teacher's cognizance of the two stages.

In general after examining the strengths and weaknesses of criterion-referenced devices, norm-referenced devices, and observation, many special educators have come to two conclusions: (1) criterion-referenced devices provide more information which facilitates programming than do norm-referenced devices, and (2) in order to give the teacher the broadest possible picture of the child, criterion-referenced assessment must be combined with clinical and/or behavioral observation.

WHAT IS OBSERVATION?

Watching and recording a child's behavior during activities which take place during the regular day—specifically observing the child's interactions with adults, peers, and materials—is referred to as observation.

Observation techniques are useful in noting the interests of the child, his use of language, patterns of adjustment, and learning characteristics. Because such techniques help in catching the subtleties missed by other types of assessment, they allow the teacher to meet the ultimate goal of the assessment process: i.e., understanding the whole child. For observation procedures and techniques to be most valuable, they must allow systematic and precise recording over a period of time so that the pattern and frequency of behavior can be determined.

The following eight procedures are representative of different types of observation techniques. The use of each procedure varies depending upon the person implementing it. For example, anecdotal accounts (No. 3) differ substantially among teachers with respect to length, specificity of content, topic, and frequency.

Note that the techniques become more structured in terms of the demands made upon the user as you move through the list.

1. Snapshots — Some teachers take pictures of children during different activities over a period of time. They then collect these snapshots and analyze the child's expressions, activities, and interactions with others.

2. Work samples — Those who use this procedure periodically select a sample of the child's work and put it in a folder. The teacher can then look back over the work and determine whether or not the child is making progress in skill development. Sometimes this technique is also used to analyze a child's feelings about himself. For example, the child draws a picture during free time. The teacher analyzes the content, composition, perspective, color choice, and size of various components in order to try to understand the child's feelings.

3. Anecdotal accounts, logs, diaries, and narratives — The teacher makes entries or jots down his observations about particular children or a group of children. He writes down what he remembers and what he thinks is important. This is usually done at a time that is convenient for the teacher: i.e., when the children are either quiet or absent.

4. Listing of activities — The teacher records the activities in which the child participates. This is done daily for some children while the teacher only makes this kind of observation periodically for other children. This technique helps the teacher decide whether a child needs to be encouraged to develop motor skills, perceptual skills, reasoning skills, language skills, or social skills.

5. Videotape recordings and audiotape recordings — A child or group of children are taped while engaging in an activity. The teacher is usually also participating in the activity and uses these devices to capture behavior so that he can analyze it at a later date. Oftentimes, the tapes are saved so comparisons can be made between tapes.

6. Standardized observation devices — These devices list the behaviors which the teacher or his designee is to observe

and record. The observation procedures are standardized and the child usually receives a score. This score is then compared to the scores of other children. Most of these devices were designed to be used with school-age children.

7. Running record — This is a systematic observation and recording procedure which requires planning and consistency. Records should be taken at several times during the day (not necessarily on the same day) and should cover a variety of activities and behaviors, which may include events of the day such as washing, toileting, eating, resting, arrival, dismissal, transition periods, story time, small group activities, individual activities, outdoor play, indoor play, etc. Behaviors such as interactions with adults and other children, adjustment to school, feelings about routines, and the child's position in the group can also be observed. The following items should be considered in making an entry in the running record:

   a. The setting (date, place, and the situation) in which the action occurred. What is the stimulus? How is the contact made? Is it purposeful?

   b. The actions of the child, the reactions of the other people involved, and the response of the child to their responses. Who makes the contact first? What happens after the initial contact?

   c. What is said to the child and by the child during the actions? Language is the recording tool and should be used thoughtfully.

   d. "Mood cues" such as gestures, voice qualities, facial expressions, and body positions that give cues to how the child felt. What special attitudes does the child reveal? How frequently does this behavior occur?

   e. The completeness of the description and its accuracy in covering the episode. The goal is to look for emerging or prevalent behavior patterns. If after reviewing the running record you identify developmental delays or extremes in behavior, a referral may be warranted. If a referral is made, then the information collected will serve as an important resource to aid in the final diagnosis by the appropriate personnel. In cases in which a referral is not made, the running record serves as a very effective way to identify problem areas which can be strengthened through classroom programming.

8. Systematic data collection — In these procedures, the teacher is observing one specific, measurable behavior at a time. Prior to the observation, the teacher decides who he is going to observe; what behavior he will observe; exactly when he will observe; and how the observation will be done. The observation should be done at the same time and same place each day. This is the most specific and structured type of observation that we have discussed. Those who use this type of observation procedure are interested in changing (increasing or decreasing) behavior or maintaining a desirable behavior. The teacher recognizes that a problem exists and tries to determine when the specific problem behavior is occurring. He then has the choice of using a time sampling procedure or a frequency count procedure to record the behavior. In time sampling there are specific recording intervals during a block of time. For example, the block of time is a twenty-minute-long lesson. The block of time is divided into thirty-second intervals, i.e., recording for thirty seconds, not recording for thirty seconds, recording again for thirty seconds and so on until the block of time is up. If the behavior occurs during a nonrecording time it is not recorded. This recording procedure can be used when you are trying to record a specific behavior for several children in a group. For example, during play period you observe one child for thirty seconds and record how many times the behavior occurs; the next recording interval you observe another child and so on until you've observed all of the children within the group. In frequency counting there are no counting intervals. You count how many times a behavior occurs either during a short specified time, or for the entire day. The results obtained from time sampling and frequency counting are recorded on a chart or graph. This is called baseline data. After the teacher looks at the baseline data, he then decides what he is going to do each time the behavior occurs. This is called intervention. The teacher continues to record (using the same recording procedure as used to obtain baseline data) in order to ascertain whether the intervention is working.

WHAT ARE PIAGETIAN DEVICES?

These devices are perhaps the most recent innovations in the assessment of young children. As the name implies, the devices are based upon Piaget's philosophy of cognitive development which is quite different from the view of those who have constructed most of the developmental and psychological assessment devices for young children. In Piaget's philosophy, development is described as the interaction of an organism (child) possessing certain competencies with the environment. The competencies are interrelated and are changed or transformed to progressively higher levels as the organism (child) interacts with his environment. The quality and level of development at one stage depends heavily upon the level of skill acquisition at an earlier time. On the other hand, those who have developed most of the developmental and psychological assessment devices take an opposing position: "...changes in the course of development are small, gradual, and are inherently unrelated to each other; change is considered to be quantitative and no a priori assumptions are made about the relationship of a given achievement to the one that follows" (Uzgiris and Hunt, 1975).

The differences in the philosophies of the two camps have resulted in substantial differences in the construction of the tests and the type of items used in the tests. There are two major differences between the two kinds of tests. One, traditional tests presume a predetermined rate of development whereas Piagetian devices are designed to investigate the effects of various encounters upon the rate of development which is not viewed as fixed. Two, traditional tests assume that competence or intelligence is based upon a unitary ability. Those who have developed the Piagetian tests, however, view competence as "...a hierarchical organization of a number of abilities and motive systems with several relatively independent branches" (Uzgiris and Hunt, 1975). Put more simply, norm- and criterion-referenced devices are concerned with ascertaining whether or not the child has a particular skill or behavior. For example, an item found in many traditional tests is, "Child visually follows object past midline. — Yes or No?" In the "Ordinal Scales of Psychological Development" by Uzgiris and Hunt the quality or level of the infant's response to the task (follows object...) is of primary concern, and consequently, five alternative behaviors, not just yes or no, are listed.

Most of the Piagetian devices developed thus far concentrate on the sensori-motor stage of development (birth to two years of age). The exception is an earlier device developed by Lavatelli (1970). These devices offer much promise to those who are concerned with accurate and relevant programming for children, programming which attempts to enable the child to develop to his full potential.

AFTER INFORMATION HAS BEEN COLLECTED, WHAT IS THE NEXT STEP IN THE ASSESSMENT PROCESS?

Interpretation of the information obtained during the collection phase is the next and last phase in the assessment process. Interpretation is the process of reviewing, analyzing, and synthesizing all of the information on the child which has been collected. There are six steps in interpretation. They are:

1. Look at the family background and other information provided by the parents about the functioning level of the child. Note circumstances and experiences that might affect the child's abilities and behavior such as socio-economic level, place of residence, birth history, opportunity for autonomy and independence commensurate with his age, cultural background, size of family, and number and identification of caregivers.

2. Keep in mind individual characteristics of the child, such as handicapping condition, age, size, bilingual or monolingual, etc.; also note characteristics which affect learning such as hyperactivity, conceptual tempo (impulsive or reflective), persistence, etc.

3. Look at the information obtained during assessment, and compare it to the information obtained in screening and diagnosis. Compare the results and look for patterns of behavior and learning. See if the results obtained by different devices and techniques are consistent or inconsistent.

4. Based upon the information, decide which objectives are the most appropriate for the child. The teacher will have to decide how much the child will be able to accomplish given his strengths and weaknesses and what steps he must go through in order to accomplish the objectives.

5. List the objectives in order of priority. How many objectives will the child be able to accomplish and which ones are the most important?

6. Based upon the child's learning characteristics and needs, what techniques and/or procedures should be used? Does the child need information presented through the visual, auditory, or tactile channels or some combination of these? Other teaching techniques and procedures to be considered are structured lessons and environment, use of interest centers, use of behavior modification techniques, routines, the use of concrete experiences and pictures, field trips, and the type and size of materials.

WHAT IS THE OUTCOME OF THE ASSESSMENT PROCESS?

A profile of the child's abilities and educational plan are the outcomes of the assessment process. The interpretation of the assessment information forms the basis for the educational plan. Many people have developed their own forms for educational plans. The following plan (Figure 2) is an example that contains the components necessary for a comprehensive plan. However, the form and plan are meaningless if the collection and interpretation of assessment information is not done systematically, thoroughly, and accurately.

Figure 2

INDIVIDUAL EDUCATIONAL PROGRAM:
TOTAL SERVICE PLAN

Date _____ Name _____ DOB _____ Age ___

Parent's Name _____ Address _____ Phone ____

School _____ Grade _____ Teacher _____

Summary of present level of
performance (language,
academic, social/emotional
physical, vocational)

Statement of long term goals: _____

Short term objectives	Specific educational or support services required	% of time	Beginning ending dates

Percent of time
in regular classroom _____

Special Placement
recommendation _____

Teacher referral _____
Educational report _____
Permission for testing _____
Psychological report _____
Placement permission _____
Special transportation
arrangements needed ____

Program placement _____

Date _____

Placement review date _____

Participants _____
Parent's Signature _____ Date _____

BIBLIOGRAPHY

Bangs, Tina E. and Garrett, Susan. *The birth-3 scale.* Houston Speech and Hearing Center, 1975.

Bluma, S., Shearer, M., Frohman, A., and Hilliard, J. *Portage guide to early education checklist.* Portage: Portage Project, 1976.

Carver, Ronald P. Two dimensions of tests. *American Psychologist,* July, 1974, *29,* no. 7.

Cohen, Dorothy and Stern, Virginia. *Observing and recording the behavior of young children.* New York: Teacher's College Press, 1972.

Cox, Richard C. Evaluative aspects of criterion-referenced measures. In W. J. Popham (ed.), *Criterion referenced measurement.* Englewood Cliffs, N.J.: Education Technology Publications, 1973.

Haeussermann, Else. *Developmental potential of preschool children.* New York: Grune and Stratton, 1958.

Hoepfner, R., Stern, C., and Nummedal, S. *Preschool/kindergarten test evaluations.* Los Angeles: UCLA Graduate School of Education, 1971.

Lillie, D. *Early childhood education: An individualized approach to developmental instruction.* Chicago: Science Research Associates, 1975.

Lavatelli, Celia S. Piaget's theory applied to an early childhood curriculum. Great Neck, N.Y.: Center for Media Development, 1970.

Moore, C. (ed.). *Preschool programs for handicapped children.* Eugene, Ore.: University of Oregon, 1974.

Popham, W. James. *Criteria referenced measurement.* Englewood Cliffs, N.J.: Educational Technology Publications, 1973.

Sanford, Anne R. *Learning accomplishment profile.* Winston-Salem, N.C.: Kaplan School Supply Co., 1975.

Sigel, Irving E. How intelligence test limit understanding of intelligence. *Merrill-Palmer Quarterly,* 1963, *9,* no. 1.

Uzgiris, Ina C. and Hunt, J. McV. *Assessment in infancy: Ordinal scales psychological development.* Urbana, Ill.: University of Illinois Press, 1975.

Weinberg, Richard A. and Wood, Frank (eds.). *Observations of pupils and teachers in mainstream and special education settings: Alternative strategies.* Minneapolis, Minn.: Leadership Training Institute/Special Education, University of Minnesota, 1975.

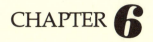

Program Evaluation
Melvin G. Moore

WHAT IS EVALUATION?

For the purposes of this book, evaluation is defined as the process of determining whether or not the educational program produced the desired results in the development of the children who entered and completed the program. The process includes *analyzing* activities against some *standards* so that *decisions* can be made about the effectiveness of the activities in helping the children reach some predetermined end.

ANALYSIS involves examining information compiled about the children; this usually includes an examination of information from measurement ACTIVITIES (diagnosis and assessment). Subjective information (e.g., feelings about the degree to which children improved) is examined only if it can be qualified in some fashion. STANDARDS are the criteria against which the measurement data are compared. The standards are frequently stated in terms of the percentage of activities accomplished by the children or the percentage of children achieving an objective. DECISION-MAKING refers to the process of interpreting the results of the analysis to determine whether the program should be maintained or modified (Paulson, 1970).

MELVIN G. MOORE is an Assistant Research Professor at Teaching Research, a Division of the Oregon State System of Higher Education. His interests include evaluation and child development.

WHAT IS THE PURPOSE OF EVALUATION?

It is to provide appropriate information when decisions are necessary. Four groups involved in service programs for children with special needs are generally faced with decision-making responsibilities which require evaluation information.

1. The *instructional staff* of the program needs frequent information about changes in the children to plan (alter or maintain) for the ongoing instructional program. The staff also needs evaluative information at the end of the program or at the end of a major segment of the program (e.g., a year) to determine if the intended outcomes were obtained; if they were not, why; and if changes in instructional strategies should be implemented in the next segment of the program.

2. The *program administrators* need evaluative information in determining whether or not to curtail, maintain, or expand single components of the program or the program as a whole.

3. The *taxpayer*, or his elected *representative*, has an "educational right" (Lessinger, 1970) to know the results of his investments. Funding agencies must be accountable for the programs that they fund.

4. *Professionals* interested in a particular intervention model will also be interested in evaluation information on changes in children. Current thinking about the ways services can be provided to all children are predicted on "copying" the skills and procedures proven valid through effective intervention, effectiveness in both methodology and results.

IS THERE MORE THAN ONE APPROACH TO EVALUATION?

Yes. The two types of evaluation generally considered most important in evaluating the effectiveness of an intervention program are *formative* and *summative* evaluation. The main difference in these two approaches lies in how the evaluative results are to be used. "Use" obviously has some bearing on how and when information is collected. With formative evaluation, results are used in planning modifications to and/or maintaining the programs for children. The phrase "summative evaluation" refers to a final accounting (usually involving a year or more) which is designed primarily to determine the overall success of a program.

Both types of evaluation are important. Summative data are necessary in showing that programs—in the long run—have been effective or ineffective. Government and other funding agencies need this kind of data for "accountability" purposes. Formative data are important, especially to teachers, in periodically making sure that programs are on course; and, if they are not, how they may be set back on course.

WHEN SHOULD PLANS FOR EVALUATION BEGIN?

Evaluation procedures should be planned at the beginning of the program—along with casefinding, screening, diagnosis, assessment, and intervention (Gallagher et al., 1973; Stoke, 1967; Stufflebeam, 1968).

SHOULD THE SERVICES OF AN OUTSIDE EVALUATOR BE OBTAINED?

The question of internal versus third-party (external) evaluation is complex, with no consistently appropriate answer. If requirements are not specified by the funding agency, it is a question with which educational personnel must deal. There are, however, a number of factors to consider when making such a decision.

Many programs have been funded that have experienced and recognized "expert" evaluators on the staff. Under such conditions, it is possible that assistance in evaluation from someone outside the project may not be desired or needed. Such projects may obtain the services of an outside evaluator, however, to assist in or react to planned evaluative procedures. For programs with personnel with little or no previous experience, outside evaluators may be hired on at least a part-time basis. In situations where the evaluator is not directly involved in program functioning, precise agreement must be achieved between the evaluator and program personnel as to what, when, and how data are to be collected, compiled, and reported.

Another factor to consider is credibility. Situations may arise in which the concealment of failures of program outcomes may be suspected by outsiders if all evaluation is internal. The employment of a third party in the evaluation process, though not totally negating the possibility of prejudiced results, tends to encourage a favorable impression of the program among outsiders.

WHAT KINDS OF PROCEDURES CAN BE USED TO EVALUATE CHILDREN'S PROGRESS?

Some evaluative procedures are case studies, experimental research designs, and normative- or criterion-referenced assessments. Procedures and instruments will vary from program to program. For some, norm-referenced devices may be useful; for others, criterion-referenced instruments may be of value. In addition, checklists, rating scales, and observational tools might be used to measure and demonstrate the progress of children.

IN ADDITION TO BEHAVIORAL CHANGE DATA, WHAT OTHER EVALUATIVE DATA SHOULD BE COLLECTED ON CHILDREN?

Certainly, for every child, a program should maintain all relevant screening, diagnostic, assessment, evaluative, and socio-demographic information. This information may include results from various psychological, medical, or educational examinations. Such data provide the program with certain behavioral criteria both for making acceptance decisions and, if necessary, for justifying the inclusion of the child in only certain aspects of the program. *This information must be kept confidential, however, and used only when appropriate in the educational process.* Although it may not play a functional role in the evaluation of children's progress during enrollment in the program, the information may be necessary in general reporting procedures, and it provides significant background and rationale data that are useful when gains are reported.

If a program is considered innovative or if it is to "demonstrate" new approaches, the program personnel are frequently requested to provide basic kinds of "cost effectiveness data." To divide the total cost of the program by the number of children in the program is a woefully inadequate method for showing cost effectiveness because it does not account for the numerous factors that affect costs. Programs should develop strategies that will allow for maintaining various line item costs (diagnostic services, instruction, transportation, equipment, etc.) for each individual child. A comprehensive analysis of cost effectiveness necessitates continual documentation of such things as attendance, frequency and extent of diagnostic services, services purchased outside the project, amount of instruction, and other items that can be shown to require expenditures of resources (human, financial, or otherwise).

With this information, program personnel can report cost effectiveness data by individual, age group, handicapped condition, or across other variables requested by program administrators and the funding agency.

Many programs have as their terminal goal placing children in more natural educational settings. Once the children are placed, however, they cease to maintain records on the degree to which the children adapt to their new environments. Consequently, it is impossible to assess why certain children "make it" in the new setting and others do not. More sensitive evaluation plans which go beyond the confines of the program would provide clearer information about why children succeed (or fail) once they have left the program and would allow modifications in existing training as necessary.

HOW CAN ALL THE DATA BE MANAGED?

It was stressed earlier that evaluation strategies should be established during the program's planning phase because evaluation activities must be both continuous and methodological; this maxim also holds true for data collection techniques. Data collection for the sake of simplicity may be divided into three basic periods: initial, interim, and ending. Data to be collected during the *initial* phases of the program include: (1) the child-centered information that is required by administrators and funding agencies, (2) pretest or program entry data that will be needed in evaluating the yearly progress of children, and (3) developmental assessments for preparing the instructional program. Throughout the provision of educational services, the *interim* period, the instructional staff will need to keep continuous data on the children's skill development in all curricular areas. Maintaining records on methods of instruction in an anecdotal or prescriptive fashion makes it possible to answer questions which may come from outsiders or staff about the effectiveness of instructional strategies. Thus, an after-the-fact accounting of teaching methods becomes unnecessary. Data to be collected toward the *end* of the program year are results from posttesting and from compiling and organizing formative data on the children for summative reporting.

Where and how the data are maintained should be determined by considering which program personnel will most often use the various data. Undoubtedly, the initial descriptive types of information should be kept in a centrally located file, perhaps in the program director's office for easy reference. Program administrators need such information as they communicate with individuals outside the program. However, instructional information should be easily accessible to teachers for their instructional planning and interaction with parents and visitors. All program staff should know where to find the various types of data that are kept on the children served by the program.

HOW SHOULD PROGRAM EFFECTIVENESS BE REPORTED?

Reporting the effectiveness of a program is as much a part of the evaluative process as collecting data. Audiences for the report should be identified and decisions should be made on how the data will be reported well in advance of the reporting.

The purpose for distributing evaluative information is to indicate to the audience the extent of program accomplishments. In preparing dissemination documents, the aim should be efficiency and understanding. Both the text and tabular data should be descriptive but concise, focusing on the essential elements of the program. Tables are essential for organizing large amounts of data and should be used where appropriate throughout the report, each effectively labeled and self-explanatory. Written sections require caution in the language employed. Any audience will resist technical jargon even if such vocabulary may add considerably to the preciseness of the message conveyed. However, points of significance should be explained as necessary and documented with facts from tables.

BIBLIOGRAPHY

Gallagher, J.; Surles, R.; and Hayes, A. *Program planning and evaluation*. Chapel Hill: Technical Assistance Development System, 1973.

Paulson, C. *A strategy for evaluation design*. Momouth, Oregon: Teaching Research, 1970.

Stoke, R. E. The countenance of educational evaluation. *Teachers College Record*, 1967, *68*, 523-540.

Stufflebeam, O. L. Toward a science of educational evaluation. *Educational Technology*, 1968, *8*, 5-12.

PART TWO

A Bibliography of Screening, Diagnosis and Assessment Instruments

CHAPTER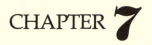

Introduction
Lee Cross

This bibliography grew from a book published by TADS in 1973 called the *Evaluation Bibliography*. The original document was compiled by Ellen Potter with the assistance of Gloria Harbin. It primarily included instruments that were being used by programs in the Handicapped Childrens Early Education Program (HCEEP).

During the years since the publication was released, many new instruments have surfaced. Most of the entries that we have added were developed by centers that were part of the HCEEP. We have made every effort to survey the HCEEP thoroughly and to include instruments which were useful for screening, diagnosis, and/or assessment as defined in the preceding chapters. Any omissions are oversights except in a few cases, particularly in the area of screening, where tests did not meet the appropriate criteria. Inclusion of an instrument within the bibliography should not be interpreted as an endorsement by TADS.

"Age, use, and performance factors" are the areas in which information is provided for each test in the matrix. Instruments have been classified according to their *primary* use (screening, diagnosis, or assessment). In most cases, instruments classified as diagnostic can be used for assessment purposes. This duality is not indicated in the matrix. Norm-referenced tests can be found under

LEE CROSS is Director of Early Childhood Education at the Frank Porter Graham Child Development Center at the University of North Carolina, Chapel Hill. Her interests include programming for preschool handicapped children and assessment.

diagnosis while criterion-referenced instruments are under *assessment*. In some cases, we have indicated a different use for an instrument than the use specified by the developer. The relabeling was necessary because of the purposes that we feel each of the activities described in this book serve. For example, we have often placed tests that were deemed screening instruments by their developers under the label of assessment when their standardization, validity, and reliability had not been established.

Test developers indicated different performance factors in describing their tests. We have used our best judgment in classifying each instrument in terms of performance factors explained below:

GROSS MOTOR.   The development of large muscle skills such as running, walking, climbing, throwing, and sitting. Body perception, static balance, dynamic balance, general body coordination, speed and agility, and endurance are the skills included in this area.

FINE MOTOR.   The development of small muscle skills such as cutting, writing, and bead stringing. Skills include finger dexterity, finger speed, hand and finger dexterity, hand and finger speed, arm and hand precision, and arm steadiness.

PERCEPTION.   The ability to attach meaning or order to incoming tactile and visual stimuli. Perception skills include sensory awareness, intrasensory integration, perceptual accuracy, figure-ground, spatial relationships, perceptual flexibility, perceptual closure, perceptual memory, and directionality.

LANGUAGE.   The systematic means of expressing and receiving information. Language skills include structural use/comprehension, attending, sounds, imitation, auditory reception, auditory memory, auditory association, word meaning, verbal expression, and manual expression.

SOCIAL.   The ability to relate to the environment and to others in a positive and meaningful way. Social skills include body awareness, self-concept development, understanding others, relationships with others, and self-help skills.

Cost and availability information is included with each annotation. Cost information may change periodically. Persons interested in further information about each test should contact the source indicated.

CHAPTER **8**

The Bibliography
Lee Cross
and Sonya Johnston

ABC Inventory (N. Adair and G. Blesch). Muskegan, MI: Research Concepts, 1965.

The *ABC Inventory* is designed to identify children aged four to six who are likely to fail in kindergarten or who are not likely to be ready for grade one. It includes items related to drawing, copying, folding, counting, memory, general information, colors, size concepts, time concepts, and the like. The *Inventory* is individually administered, paced, and takes about nine minutes to give. No special training is needed to administer the questionnaire. Raw scores are related to "ready ages," which are highly correlated with mental ages (*Stanford-Binet*). Reliability studies consisted of testing the means of two comparable groups who took the *Inventory* in 1962 and in 1964. Studies of the relationships between those students who scored below certain cutting scores and those who failed in kindergarten or the first grade are reported.

Available from: Research Concepts
1368 E. Airport Rd.
Muskegan, MI 49441

or

Educational Studies and Development
1357 Forrest Park Rd.
Muskegan, MI 49441

Cost: $ 5.90 50 copies
$ 9.40 100 copies
$37.90 500 copies

SONYA JOHNSTON is Research Associate at the Technical Assistance Development System in Chapel Hill. Her interests include curriculum and technical assistance training.

Adaptive Behavior Scales (N. Nihira, R. Foster, M. Shellhas, and H. Leland). Washington: American Association on Mental Deficiency, 1974.

The *Adaptive Behavior Scale* is an informant-interview behavior-rating scale for mentally retarded and emotionally maladjusted individuals. It provides information on such individuals' effectiveness in coping with the natural social demands of their environments. The *Scale* assesses the important area of how independent the individual is able to be. There are two forms of the *Scale*; the one reported here is for children twelve years of age or younger. Since some items are not appropriate for very young children, a list of items omitted for children under five is given on each page. Part I of the test taps ten behavior domains: independent functioning, physical development, economic activity, language development, number and time concept, domestic duties, self-direction, responsibilities, and socialization. Part II provides information on maladaptive behavior, such as violent and destructive behavior, untrustworthy behavior, inappropriate interpersonal manners, and hyperactive tendencies. Points are given for each response to yield scores which may be compared with scores from institutional populations. However, unscored responses are also informative.

Available from: American Association of Mental Deficiency
5201 Connecticut Avenue, N.W.
Washington, DC 20015

Cost: $1.00 Scale (100 for $50)
$5.00 Manual (ten for $40)

Assessment by Behavior Rating (E. Sharp). Tucson: University of Arizona, 1975.

The *Assessment by Behavior Rating* (ABR) was developed for use by early education programs, like Head Start, serving two- through four-year-old children. It is a criterion-referenced instrument based on normative assessment. Baseline information is provided in four areas of growth and development: physical, self-help, language, and social. The language section has its theoretical foundation in Samuel A. Kirk's model of the communication process.

The two major objectives of the instrument are: (1) to indicate strengths, weaknesses, or average development in physical skills, self-help skills, language skills, and social skills; and (2) to indicate a child's developmental age in each of the four areas assessed.

The ABR can be used as a screening instrument by staff who have a good background in the sequential patterns of development, and it can be used to group children by ability level.

The *Manual for the Assessment by Behavior Rating* includes a description of the scale, a statement about its purpose, and directions for use. It provides suggested activities for each item on the scale as well as the criteria for rating.

Available from: Dr. Elizabeth T. Sharp
Department of Special Education
College of Education

University of Arizona
Tucson, AZ 85721

Cost: $2.50

Assessment-Programming Guide for Infants and Preschoolers (W. Umansky). Columbus: Developmental Services, Inc., 1974

This new edition of the *Assessment-Programming Guide for Infants and Preschoolers*, formerly available as the *Developmental Evaluation and Programming Guide* (Savage, 1972), encompasses several major changes that standardize its use in programs for normal and handicapped children, 0-72 months. The contents have been rearranged and much of the language has been clarified.

The contents of the manual, including developmental scales and accompanying appendices, have two purposes: (1) to aid in determining the needs of a child through systematic observation, and (2) to provide guidelines and direction in planning a program to the child's specific needs.

The manual is compiled to reflect a child's level of development in six areas: motor, perceptual-motor, language, self-help, social-personal. "Academic" was added to reflect an orientation toward education of the child. When an item is of relative importance to several areas, it is listed under each of the appropriate areas.

Within each developmental area, skills are grouped by the age at which they appear in a majority of the population. Within each category, items are listed in approximate order of appearance in a child's repertoire. Items have been worked to maximize objectivity of interpretation between evaluators.

Familiarity with the development scales and evaluation procedures outlined is the minimal requirement for a teacher to use the manual. Complete evaluation of a child may take several weeks since items are planned for spontaneous exhibition rather than for a structured test situation; however, the evaluator may wish to plan activities which maximize the opportunities for specific behaviors to be observed.

The information generated through the use of this manual provides a meaningful tool to communicate program goals and strategies to the parents.

Available from: Developmental Services, Inc.
1541 Hutchins Avenue
Columbus, IN 47201
(812) 372-0259

Cost: $2.50

Auditory Discrimination Test (J. Wepman). Los Angeles: Western Psychological Services, 1973.

This test requires about five minutes to administer and presents matched words which the child is asked to indicate as being the same or different. Test results are interpreted in terms of either adequate or inadequate development of auditory discrimination, with cut-off points given starting at age five. The test lacks the sophistication of the *Golden-Fristoe-Woodcock*, but appears to be a simple and efficient instrument for limited purposes.

Available from: Western Psychological Services
Publishers and Distributors
12301 Wilshire Blvd.
Los Angeles, CA 90025

Cost: $9.50 Kit (includes 40 LR-3A Tests, 20 IA Forms, 20 IIA Forms, and 1 LR-3B Manual)
$6.00 1 Package (includes 25 LR-3A Tests and either 25 IA or IIA Forms)
$5.00 2-19 Packages
$4.00 20+ Packages
$2.00 1 LR-3B Manual

Basic Concept Inventory (S. Engelmann). Chicago: Follett Publishing Company, 1967.

The *Basic Concept Inventory* provides a broad checklist of basic concepts that are involved in new learning situations and are used in explanations and instructions in first grade. It is primarily intended for culturally disadvantaged preschool and kindergarten children, slow learners, emotionally disturbed children, and mentally retarded children. Although designed for young children, it may be given to children aged three to ten. The *Inventory* is criterion-referenced and uses basic concepts, sentence repetition and comprehension, and pattern-awareness tasks. It is individually administered, paced, and requires about twenty minutes. If the *Inventory* is to be used as a basis for remedial instruction, it may be given by the classroom teacher. If, however, it is to be used diagnostically as the basis for special treatment or special placement, a trained examiner should administer the instrument. Reliability and validity studies are reported to be in progress.

Available from: Follett Publishing Company
1010 W. Washington Blvd.
Chicago, IL 60607

Cost: $ 4.95 Package of fifteen booklets (3700 code number)
$30.00 Package of 100 booklets, one manual & one set of cards (3703)
$ 3.30 Picture cards, set of nine (3701)
$ 3.30 Manual (3702)

Bayley Scales of Infant Development (N. Bayley). Atlanta: The Psychological Corporation, 1969.

The *Bayley Scales of Infant Development* assess developmental status in infants from birth to thirty months of age. The Mental Scale (163 items) measures sensory-perceptual acuities and discriminations; early acquisition of object constancy and memory, learning, and problem-solving ability; vocalizations and the beginning of verbal communication; and early evidence of the ability to form generalizations and classifications. The Motor Scale (81 items) measures the degree of control of the body, coordination of the large muscles, and finer manipulatory skills of the hands and fingers. Each of these items has an age placement to the nearest one-tenth of a month and an age range. The last part of the test is an Infant Behavior Record, consisting of thirty ratings, which is completed by the examiner after the Scales have been administered on the basis of his observation. It deals with social orientation, emotional variables, object relations, motivational variables, activity, reactivity, sensory areas of interest displayed, and general evaluations. Some props are needed. A kit of the materials used for the norming groups is available. The test is untimed (although certain items are timed) and individually administered. Training is needed. The mother (or mother substitute) is present during the test. Average testing time for the Mental and Motor Scales is forty-five minutes with about ten percent of the cases requiring seventy-five minutes or more. Raw scores may be converted to Mental Development and Motor Development indices, scores standardized by age with a mean of 100 and standard deviation of sixteen, or to mental ages. Evidence of face validity is presented. Split-half, test-retest, tester-observer reliabilities, and correlations with *Stanford-Binet* I.Q.'s for sample members aged twenty-four, twenty-seven, and thirty months are reported.

Available from: The Psychological Corporation
1372 Peachtree Street, N.E.
Atlanta, GA 30309

Cost: $98.00 Complete set (manual, record forms (twenty-five each) case)

The Bayley Scales of Infant Development: Modifications for Youngsters with Handicapped Conditions (H. Hoffman). Commack, NY: Suffolk Rehabilitation Center, 1974

The *Modification*, which is administered as a second level test when a psychologist deems it appropriate, is designed to assess cognitive development in handicapped babies, two to thirty months, by circumventing the effects of their physical limitations.

An initial score is determined by the standard *Bayley*. A second score is achieved by modifying standard testing procedures through changes in positioning of the child, and/or additional team members or parents participating in the testing, and/or the use of alternative equipment which has physical qualities that allow the handicapped child to demonstrate his understanding of the task required.

Administration time for the modification requires from ten minutes to one and one-half hours for one or two sessions.

Available from: TMA Outreach Program
Suffolk Rehabilitation Center
159 Indian Head Road
Commack, NY 11725

Cost: $.13 Postage

Beery-Buktenica Developmental Test of Visual-motor Integration (K. Beery and N. Buktenica). Chicago: Follett Educational Corporation, 1967.

This test assesses the degree to which visual perception and motor behavior are integrated. It consists of a series of twenty-four geometric forms which the subject is asked to copy without erasures or corrections. The *Test* is for ages two to fifteen years, and scores provide a visual-motor integration-age equivalent. According to Beery, there are five levels of visual-motor integration. It is considered a fairly complete test of visual-motor functioning in young children.

Available from: Follett Publishing Company
1010 W. Washington Blvd.
Chicago, IL 60607

Cost: Short Form
$ 6.90 Package of fifteen (#3736)
$45.00 Package of 100 (#3737)
$ 5.40 Administration scoring manual (#3731)
$ 6.57 Monograph and stimulus cards (#3732)
$24.00 Assessment workshops (#3733)
$ 2.10 Specimen set (#3735)

Behavioral Development Profile (M. Donahue, J. Montgomery, A. Keiser, V. Roecker, and L. Smith). Marshalltown, IA: Marshalltown Project, 1975

The *Behavioral Development Profile* is designed to measure the development of handicapped and culturally deprived children ages zero through six and to facilitate individualized teaching of preschool children within the home setting.

The items are based upon normal child development; that is, they are taken from normative sources. The *Profile* consists of behavioral skills specifically stated and divided into three scales: Communication, Motor, and Social. The items within each category are arranged according to age. This is a criterion-referenced device designed to measure the progress of each child in months.

The instrument is used with a score sheet and Behavioral Prescription Guides. The Guides list behavioral objectives and the activities to accomplish each objective in sequential steps. There are objectives for each of the skills measured in the *Profile*.

The results from the *Profile* are used to ascertain the level of development along with strengths and weaknesses. The person who is working with the child then uses this information to set objectives and choose strategies for accomplishing those objectives.

Available from: Marshalltown Project
507 East Anson
Marshalltown, IA 50158

Cost: $3.00

Bender Motor Gestalt Test (L. Bender). Albany: American Orthopsychiatric Association, 1938.

The *Bender Gestalt Test* consists of eight designs which are copied by the child under standard conditions and scored for specific errors in reproduction. It is a clinical device used to detect visual perceptual difficulties and the possible presence of brain damage. It is for individuals aged four years and up. It is described as "a maturational test of visual-motor gestalt function in children, to explore retardation, regression, loss of function and organic brain defects, and personality deviations." Its major use is as a diagnostic instrument. Many scoring schemes are available, but all lack substantial population norms.

Available from: American Orthopsychiatric Association
Sales Office
49 Sheridan Avenue
Albany, NY 12210

Cost: $8.50 Visual Motor Gestalt Test and Clinical Uses
$3.00 Bender Visual Motor Gestalt Test: Cards and Manual of Instruction.

Birth-3 Scale (T. Bangs and S. Garrett). Houston: Houston Speech and Hearing Center, 1975.

This instrument was developed to provide baseline data for habilitation and rehabilitation procedures for those children from birth to three who were referred to the Houston Speech and Hearing Center. There are ninety items arranged according to age in six-month intervals. Alternate items have been included for standardization purposes. It is recommended that a case history of the examiner's choice be used to provide additional information.

The instrument is constructed so that it can be used and interpreted by those not specifically trained in psychometrics. The methods for scoring each item are clearly stated. The materials for the scale can be taken from standardized tests or the mother can choose the materials. The authors feel this is the first step in the development of a culture-free test.

Standardization procedures are currently in progress. The scores from the test are supposed to indicate the present developmental level of the child. The *Scale* can also be used in pre-post fashion.

Available from: Speech and Hearing Institute
University of Texas
Health Science Center at Houston
1343 Meursund Avenue
Houston, TX 77035

Cost: $5.00

Boehm Test of Basic Concepts or BTBC (A. E. Boehm). Atlanta: The Psychological Corporation, 1971.

This test measures mastery of concepts considered necessary for achievement in the first years of school. It is appropriate for grades K-2. Pictorial multiple-choice items check concepts of quantity and number, space (location, direction, orientation, dimension), time, and miscellaneous. BTBC is group-administered and paced. Administration time is fifteen to twenty minutes for each of two test booklets. The *Test* may be given in one or two sessions depending upon age and attention span. Testing in small groups (eight to twelve) or using assistants is helpful with younger children. No special training is needed to administer the *Test*. Percentile norms by grade and by socio-economic level are available. Split-half reliabilities are reported. Content validity is inferred from the item selection procedures. No other validity data are reported.

Available from: The Psychological Corporation
1372 Peachtree Street, N.E.
Atlanta, GA 30309

Cost: $6.75 Booklets (thirty/pkg.)
$ .60 per copy

Burks Behavior Rating Scales (H. Burks). Huntington Beach: Arden Press, 1969.

The *Burks Behavior Rating Scale* is a means by which teachers or untrained individuals can record behavioral or learning disorders that are indicative of organic brain dysfunction. It consists of thirty items: e.g., "hyperactive and restless," "cries often and easily," "explosive and unpredictable behavior," "often tells bizarre stories." The teacher can rate each of these items on a five-point scale from "have not noticed this behavior at all" to "have noticed this behavior to a very large degree" for each child. The scale is designed for grades one through six.

Available from: Arden Press
8331 Alvarado
Huntington Beach, CA 92646

Cost: $5.25 Pkg. of twenty-five
$4.50 Manual
$2.95 Teacher's manual

2 forms: Elementary - Secondary
Preschool - Kindergarten

Bzoch-League Receptive-Expressive Emergent Language Scale (K. P. Bzoch and R. League). Tallahassee: Anhinga Press, 1971.

This scale aids the evaluator in investigating emerging expressive and receptive language skills in very young children (birth through three years) and in detecting handicaps in language acquisition. The *Scale* contains items for specific age periods, half of which deal with receptive language and half of which deal with expressive language. There are six items for each month for the first year, six items for each two-month interval for the second year, and six items for each four-month period for the third year. The *Scale* can usually be completed by an interview with the mother or principal caretaker, although occasionally direct observation is necessary. The test yields a receptive language age, expressive language age, and combined language age. All of these results can also be expressed as language quotients. The manual includes an explanation of the conceptualizations of language acquisition that dictated the *Scale's* construction.

Available from: Anhinga Press
Route 2, Box 153
Tallahassee, FL 32301

Cost: $9.75 (instructional manual)
$6.75 (twenty-five forms)
$1.00 discount for purchasing manual and forms together

Cain Levine Social Competency Scale (L. F. Cain, S. Levine, and F. F. Elzey). Palo Alto: Consulting Psychologists Press, 1963.

The *Cain Levine Social Competency Scale* measures the social competence of trainable mentally retarded children aged five to thirteen. The *Scale* is divided into four subscales: self-help (manipulative and motor skills), initiative (self-directedness), social skills (interpersonal relationships), and communication (understandability). Many of the items deal with skills which would be deemed maturational in the normal child. The *Scale* consists of forty-four items and is completed by interviewing a person who has had considerable opportunity to observe the child. The interviewer must have some skill in the task in order to obtain accurate responses from the respondent. Chronological age percentile norms for trainable mentally retarded children, for the total score, and for the four subscores are available. Odd-even and test-retest reliabilities are reported. No validity studies were available for review.

Available from: Consulting Psychologists Press
577 College Avenue
Palo Alto, CA 94306

Cost: $ 1.75 Specimen set (manual and test book)
$ 1.00 Manual
$ 4.50 Pkg. of twenty-five test booklets
$16.50 100 test booklets
$75.00 500 test booklets

California Preschool Social Competency Scale or CPSCS (S. Levine, F. F. Elzey, and M. Lewis). Palo Alto: Consulting Psychologists Press, 1969.

The *California Preschool Social Competency Scale* is designed to measure the adequacy of interpersonal behavior and the degree of assumption of social responsibility in children of ages two to five. The behaviors included are situational in nature and were selected in terms of common cultural expectations to represent basic competencies to be developed in the process of socialization. Each item contains four descriptive statements, posed in behavioral terms, representing varying degrees of competency. The CPSCS contains thirty items designed to be rated by a classroom teacher. The nature of the items requires the rater to have had considerable opportunity to observe the child in a variety of situations. Age percentile norms by occupational level and total sample are available. Interrater reliabilities are reported.

Available from: Consulting Psychologists Press
577 College Avenue
Palo Alto, CA 94306

Cost: $ 1.50 Specimen set (manual and test booklet)
$ 1.25 Manual
$ 4.00 Pkg. of twenty-five test booklets
$14.00 100 test booklets
$65.00 500 test booklets

Callier-Azusa Scales (R. Stillman, ed.). Dallas: Callier Center for Communications Disorders, University of Texas at Dallas, 1975.

The *Callier-Azusa Scale* is a developmental scale designed specifically to aid in the assessment and development of an individualized program for deaf-blind and multihandicapped children. The *Callier-Azusa Scale* is composed of subscales in five areas: motor development, perceptual development, daily living skills, language development, and socialization. Each subscale is made up of sequential steps describing developmental milestones. Some steps are divided into two or more items. Space is provided for comments by the teacher. The *Scale* is designed to be comprehensive particularly at the lower developmental levels. Complete reliability information is available from the editor.

Available from: Callier Center for Communications Disorders
University of Texas/Dallas
1966 Inwood Road
Dallas, TX 75235

Cost: $3.00

Carolina Developmental Profile (D. L. Lillie). Winston-Salem, N.C.: Kaplan School Supply, 1976.

The *Carolina Developmental Profile* is a criterion-referenced checklist of skills expected of children aged two to five years. The skills are in five areas: fine motor, gross motor, perceptual reasoning, receptive language, and expressive language. The purpose of the *Profile* is to expose those areas in which the child is weak so that the teacher may plan instructional objectives that are appropriate for him. Each task is classified into a subcategory (for example, fine motor includes finger flexibility, arm and hand precision, and hand and finger dexterity). For each task, there is a task description, developmental age, needed materials, and criteria for passing. The *Profile* is presently an experimental edition which is not in final form.

Available from: Kaplan School Supply
600 Jonestown Road
Winston-Salem, NC 27103

Cost: $ .75 each
$15.00 set of twenty-five

Cassel Developmental Record (R. N. Cassel). Jacksonville: Psychologists and Educators, 1954.

The *Cassel Developmental Record* is essentially a record form on which many developmental profiles may be plotted on the same individual at different ages. Profiles span the dimensions of chronological age, physiological development, emotional development, psycho-sexual development, intellectual development, social development, and educational development—providing an average total developmental age. Chronological ages are from birth to old age. The author suggests using objective test data (from such instruments as the *Vineland* and *Gesell Scales*) when they are available. If test data are not available, the profiles do provide guidelines. The author also suggests that the profile be used for young children, where developmental factors may determine educational objectives, and that it become a part of the child's cumulative file.

Available from: Psychologists and Educators, Inc.
211 W. State
Jacksonville, IL 62650

Cost: $7.50 + $1.00 postage Specimen set (manual and one form)
$6.25 each pkg. (twenty-five forms)

Cattell Infant Intelligence Scale (P. Cattell). Atlanta: The Psychological Corporation, 1940.

This instrument measures intelligence in children from age two months to two-and-a-half years. The *Scale* has five items and one or two alternate items for each age level. The levels are at one-month intervals from two to twelve months of age, two-month intervals from twelve to twenty-four months, and three-month intervals from twenty-four to thirty months. The score obtained is the child's mental age. A number of props are needed. The test is untimed and individually administered by a person with a sound background in child psychology, including mental testing of children and a nursery school training course. Testing time is twenty to forty minutes. Item response rates for various ages of infants are reported. Spearman-Brown reliabilities and predictive validities with *Stanford-Binet* scores (thirty-six months) are available.

Available from: The Psychological Corporation
1372 Peachtree Street, N.E.
Atlanta, GA 30309

Cost: $96.00 Complete set

Children's Self-Social Constructs Test (R. Ziller, B. Long, and E. Henderson). Gainesville: Robert Ziller, 1973.

The test is a measure of self-concept. The preschool test (ages three to eight years) is individually administered and untimed and takes about ten minutes. The preschool form measures dependency, esteem, realism color, and realism size. A child is required to select a circle, draw a circle, or paste a circle to represent himself or someone else. Psychometric data are available. Further information is given in the *ERIC Head Start Test Collection Self Concept Bibliography*.

Available from: Dr. Robert Ziller
Department of Psychology
University of Florida
Gainesville, FL 32601

Cost: $.13 Postage

CIRCUS (A. Scarvia, G. Bogatz, T. Draper, A. Jungeblut, G. Sedwell, W. Ward, and A. Yates). Princeton: ETS, 1974.

Circus is designed to measure the instructional needs of individual children, aged four to six years, so that classroom activities can be planned to meet each child's needs. *Circus* is a collection of seventeen instruments. There are five measures of language development. There are also measures of qualitative understanding, visual discrimination, perceptual motor coordination, letter and numeral recognition and discrimination, sound discrimination, visual and associative memory, and problem solving. Three instruments which must be completed by the teacher are also included: one of children's classroom activities, one of their test-taking behavior, and a questionnaire about the children's educational environment. These instruments may be administered to groups of children by teachers or paraprofessionals with no special training. Users may choose from the seventeen measures those which they think are most appropriate. There is a teacher's manual for each instrument and a corresponding pupil's booklet in which the child marks his response.

Circus users have a choice of three scoring arrangements, all of which yield both numerical scores and sentence reports describing children's performance: (1) test booklets are sent to ETS for scoring and reporting; (2) children's responses are transcribed onto the *Circus* Response Record which ETS scores and reports; or (3) all booklets are scored locally by hand with detailed instructions provided by ETS for scoring and interpreting each measure.

Available from: Circus
Box 2814
Princeton, NJ 08540

Cost: $ 5.00 Specimen set
$12.50 Core package - (consists of Listen to the Story, How Much and How Many, Circus Behavior Inventory Educational Environment Questionnaire, plus one additional measure for ten children)
$ 3.75 Most other measures (pkg. of ten)

Classroom Screening (N. Giessman, S. Hering, S. Issacson, A. Fazie, and C. Tarchin). Piedmont: Circle Preschool, 1975.

This assessment device assists the classroom teacher in obtaining a class profile of skills in six areas of child development: gross motor, fine motor, self-help, social-emotional, cognitive, and language. These skills usually emerge between the years of two-and-a-half and five and are important for a child's involvement in a school program. The profile indicates where the majority of the class is functioning so that a curriculum at the children's levels can be planned.

For a half-hour a day, over a two-week period, at the beginning of the school year, the teacher observes and records these skills whenever possible during the daily schedule. To increase the possibility of their occurrence, the various tasks in each particular area of this device have been written as lesson plans for small groups.

Available from: Circle Preschool
9 Lake Avenue
Piedmont, CA 94611

Cost: $1.00

Communicative Evaluation Chart (R. Anderson, M. Miles, and P. Matheny). Cambridge: Educators Publishing Service, Inc., 1963.

This chart for children from infancy to five years of age is a screening device that gives an impression of the child's overall abilities. From twelve to twenty-five items are given for the ages of three months, six months, nine months, one year, one and one-half years, two years, three years, four years, and five years. Half the items deal with the development and comprehension of language as a communicative tool, while the other half deal with physical growth and development, motor coordination, and visual-motor responses. Some items can be reported, while others require a response from the child. This is essentially a checklist of items categorized by age. Norms are based on other tests.

Available from: Educators Publishing Services, Inc.
75 Maulton Street
Cambridge, MA 01238

Cost: $.25 each, under 100 (Catalog number 213)
$.20 each, over 100 (Catalog number 213)

Comprehensive Early Education Profile (K. F. King, L. Joyner, M. Smith, A. Thompson, M. Meredith, L. Bishop, J. Newquist, L. Brewer, Q. I. Davis). Birmingham: Comprehensive Early Education Program, 1975.

The *Comprehensive Early Education Profile* (CEEP) is designed to screen children, birth through seven years of age, in nine areas of development: auditory, comprehension, verbal communication, cognitive number, cognitive reading, gross motor, fine motor, creativity, and adaptive behavior.

The CEEP screening instrument has three purposes. First, it assists in the identification of children with developmental problems: that is, children who will have a high probability of encountering difficulties in their development and will need further assistance. Second, it identifies specific areas of a child's development which warrant more in-depth investigation. Third, it helps in the development of an individual curriculum based on the child's responses to the CEEP screening instrument.

Standardization is in process on approximately 9,000 Head Start children screened in October and November, 1975.

Available from: Comprehensive Early Education Program
1720 7th Avenue South
Birmingham, AL 35294

Cost: $7.00 Manual

Comprehensive Identification Process (R. R. Zehrbach). Bensenville: Scholastic Testing Service, 1975.

The *Comprehensive Identification Process* (CIP) was developed to facilitate the casefinding and screening of children between the ages of two-and-a-half and five-and-a-half. CIP can be administered in thirty to forty minutes per child. Cost of materials for administration is $.56 per child. The CIP screens children in eight areas: cognitive-verbal, fine motor, gross motor, speech and expressive language, social/affective, hearing, vision, and medical history. In addition, CIP suggests a process for locating children for screening. Children are screened by a team of professionals and paraprofessionals.

Support data on more than 1,000 children indicate a high degree of efficiency in identifying children in need of special assistance. Items on the CIP were taken from standardized instruments and have been restandardized on 1,000 children.

Available from: Scholastic Testing Service
480 Meyer Road
Bensenville, IL 60106

Cost: $54.50 Kit

Criterion-Referenced Placement Tests. Logan, UT: Mapps Project, 1975.

The *Criterion-Referenced Placement Tests* were developed to assess children, ages zero to five years, to determine entry level skills in receptive language, expressive language, and motor development. The instruments are used in conjunction with the Curriculum and Monitoring System (CAMS), but they may be used alone. They may be used on a pre- and posttest basis to measure gain.

The test items were developed from sequenced curriculum objectives in the three areas (receptive and expressive language and motor development) and only take twenty-five minutes each to administer by anyone who has experience in working with young children.

Available from: Glendon Casto
MAPPS Project
Exceptional Child Center
Utah State University
Logan, UT 84322

Cost: $3.50 per test (may be duplicated)

Del Rio Language Screening Test (A. Toronto, D. Leverman). Austin: National Educational Laboratory Publishers, Inc., 1975.

The First Chance Early Education Program of the San Felipe Del Rio Consolidated Independent School District in Del Rio, Texas, has developed the *Del Rio Language Screening Test* to fulfill the increasing need of special education programs in the Southwest for a valid language screening instrument in both Spanish and English. The test rapidly identifies children whose language skills are inappropriate for their age, language, and background.

The test consists of five separate subtests, each of which may be used alone or combined with other subtests. The subtests are used diagnostically in Del Rio.

Standardization of the *Del Rio Language Screening Test* was completed with 384 children between the ages of three years and six-years-eleven-months.

It is appropriate for three major groups of children:

1. English-speaking Anglo Americans
2. Predominantly Spanish-speaking Mexican-American Children
3. Predominantly English-speaking Mexican-American Children

Validity and reliability have been established.

Available from: National Educational Publishers, Inc.
Post Office Box 1003
Austin, TX 78767

Cost: $6.00

Detroit Tests of Learning Aptitude (H. J. Baker and B. Leland). Indianapolis: Bobbs-Merrill Company Inc., 1958.

The *Detroit Tests of Learning Aptitude* is a series of nineteen subtests designed to measure abilities in reasoning and comprehension, practical judgment, verbal ability, time and space relationships, number ability, auditory attentive ability, visual attentive ability, and motor ability. The examiner selects a number of subtests (usually from nine to thirteen) appropriate to the subject. Guidelines are provided. The range of mental ages measured is three to nineteen years. Six subtests are recommended for the preschool age level. The authors also explain which subtests may be used for individuals who are visually impaired, hearing impaired, cerebral palsied, speech impaired, or who have a foreign language handicap. They report that the test is suitable for use with mentally retarded children. The *Tests* yield a general mental age as well as subtest mental ages. It was standardized on pupils in the Detroit Public Schools, a population typical of large metropolitan cities.

Available from: Bobbs-Merrill Company, Inc.
Test Division
4300 W., 62nd Street
Indianapolis, IN 46268

Cost: $9.85 Sample packet
$3.95 Book of pictoral material 1958
$5.30 Examiner's handbook (eight record forms) 1967
$6.95 Pupil record (thirty-five/pkg.) 1963
$1.95 Examiner's supplement (bibliography) 1968
$2.00 Professional handbook (Interpretation of *Tests*) 1975

Developmental Indicators for the Assessment of Learning (C. Mardell, D. Goldenberg). Highland Park, IL: DIAL Inc., 1975

Developmental Indicators for the Assessment of Learning (DIAL) is a prekindergarten screening instrument for identifying children with potential learning problems. The instrument screens children in four developmental skill areas: gross motor, fine motor, concepts, and communication. Each skill area contains seven items. DIAL is appropriate for children aged two-and-a-half to five-and-a-half and costs an average of seventy-five cents per child. Six to eight children may be screened in an hour. The screening takes twenty to thirty minutes per child and is individually administered by a five-man team of professionals and/or paraprofessionals. The screening area is arranged into four screening stations plus a play and registration area with an adult operating each station. DIAL is not a diagnostic instrument and should not be used as a basis for placement. Cut-off points are provided for boys and girls at three-month intervals. Results can be used to indicate which children are "OK," those that need to be rescreened, and those that need a diagnostic evaluation. DIAL was standardized on a stratified sample of 4,356 children. Validity and reliability have been established.

Available from: DIAL Inc.
Box 911
Highland Park, IL 60035

Cost: $99.00 (Includes manual, score sheet, and most materials)

Developmental Profile (G. Alpern and T. Boll). Indianapolis: Psychological Development Publications, 1972.

The *Developmental Profile* was designed to provide an efficient and accurate instrument which multidimensionally measures the development of children six months to twelve years of age. It is meant to be used as a screening device but contains enough information to be used in programming as well.

There are 217 items arranged by age into five scales. It can be administered in about thirty to forty minutes. The instrument was constructed so that it could be used and interpreted by people not specifically trained in psychometrics. It can be self-taught by professionals trained in testing. Others may require instruction and supervision.

The instrument was designed to use interview technique, but one can also administer the items if desirable or necessary.

The authors report studies that indicate construct and face validity of the instrument. They also report high scorer, reporter, test-retest reliability. Correlational studies have been done on the physical and academic scales but have not been done on the other three scales.

Available from: Psychological Development Publications
7150 Lakeside Drive
Indianapolis, IN 46278

Cost: $9.85 Interviewing set (manual, form 474, and ten profile and scoring forms)
$9.25 Manual and form 474
$4.10 Profile and scoring forms (pkg. of twenty-five)

Developmental Therapy Objective Rating Form or DTORF (M. Wood). Baltimore: University Park Press, 1972.

The DTORF records developmental milestones already mastered, provides criteria for grouping, provides a basis for therapeutic program planning (activities, techniques, and materials), and provides a basis for program evaluation for each child.

The 144 objectives are grouped into four areas: behavior, communication, socialization, and academics. The rating form is only a short-hand version of the complete list of objectives, each of which is accompanied by examples of mastery.

Taking only thirty-sixty minutes to administer, the DTORF is completed by the treatment team staff and other staff members who have worked closely enough with the child to ascertain his mastery of selected objectives at the middle (five weeks) and end (ten weeks) of each treatment period. The ten-weeks rating provides major focus objectives for the beginning of the next ten-weeks treatment period.

Every DTORF rating for each child in treatment classes is summarized on a DTORF Summary Form which shows ratings over time. The Short DTORF Summary is used to quantify progress in the treatment program.

The complete DTORF is contained in *The Rutland Center Model for Treating Emotionally Disturbed Children.*

Available from: The Technical Assistance Office
698 No. Pope Street
Athens, GA 30601

Cost: $5.00

or: *Developmental Therapy*, edited by Mary M. Wood

Available from: University Park Press
Chamber of Commerce Building
Baltimore, MD 21202

Cost: $9.75

The Early Intervention Developmental Profile and *Developmental Screening of Handicapped Infants: A Manual* (D. B. D'Eugenio and S. Rogers). Ann Arbor: Early Intervention Project for Handicapped Infants and Young Children, 1975.

These materials were designed to supplement the diagnostic data provided by standardized testing instruments. The *Profile* assesses children between birth and thirty-six months in language, gross motor, fine motor, social/emotional self-care, and cognitive development. Major milestones for each area of development are presented in three-month intervals. The *Profile* is designed to be administered by an interdisciplinary team of trained professionals (a psychologist or special educator, an occupation and/or a physical therapist, and a speech therapist) and can be done in forty-five minutes or less. Each *Profile* can be used four times to allow the evaluators and parents to see the child's progress. The *Manual* provides administration and scoring criteria.

Available from: The University of Michigan
Publications Distribution Service
615 East University
Ann Arbor, MI 48109

Cost: $ 3.75 for one manual and one profile (code 00952)
$ 2.50 for one profile (code 00453)
$15.00 for a package of ten profiles (code 00953)

Eliot-Pearson Screening Profile (S. J. Meisels, M. S. Wiske). Medford: Tufts University, 1976.

The *Eliot-Pearson Screening Profile* (EPSP) is designed to provide a brief and easy developmental survey of the perceptual, motor, and language development of children aged four-and-a-half to five-and-a-half. The survey takes approximately fifteen minutes to administer. Teachers and students can be trained to administer the EPSP. The instrument requires further diagnosis to identify specific problem areas and to devise appropriate educational prescriptions. The EPSP was developed for use in the Sommerville Early Screening Program which, like EPSP, includes a parent questionnaire, medical evaluation, and hearing and vision testing. The EPSP has been trial tested on more than 2,000 children. A number of test items have been taken from standardized instruments; thus there is high individual item reliability. However, reliability and validity measures are still incomplete.

Available from: Samuel J. Meisels
Eliot-Pearson Department of Child Study
Tufts University
Medford, MA 02155

Cost: $1.00 for ten manuals and ten score sheets

EMI Assessment Scale, Field Test Version (W. B. Elder). Charlottesville: Education for Multihandicapped Infants, 1975.

The *EMI Assessment Scale* is a method of assessing an infant's achievement of minibehavioral milestones in the areas of gross motor, fine motor, socialization, cognition, and language development. The tool is designed for diagnostic-prescriptive teaching programs for infants aged one to twenty-four months.

In each of the behavioral areas, three behaviors for each month of development are rated (0 = not in repertoire, - = emerging, + = constant in repertoire) by a teacher or nurse practitioner who observes the infant in structured tasks. Sequencing of behaviors, based on norms from standardized instruments, allows for ordinal scoring and comparative data. When scoring for comparative purposes (individual or group) is required, the *EMI Assessment Scale Manual* should be consulted.

Available from: Education for Multihandicapped Infants
Box 232
Charlottesville, VA 22901

Cost: $1.00

Fluharty Preschool Language Screening Test (R. Weiss). Boulder, CO: INREAL Project, 1975.

> The purpose of the *Fluharty Preschool Language Screening Test* (INREAL edition) is to identify language handicapped preschool children, three to six years of age, by assessing their linguistic skills (in the areas of phonology, semantics and syntax) in an easily administered, rapid screening (ten minutes).
>
> The speech pathologist administers the three-part test. In Part I, identification responses, through the use of familiar objects and articulation (phonology), are checked. In Part II, receptive language is checked using commands (syntax). In Part III, expressive language is checked using pictures (syntax).
>
> This test with norms and cut-off scores has been verified against a diagnostic battery that includes the ITPA, Peabody, TACL, and DSS.

> Available from: INREAL Project
> Department of Communication Disorders
> University of Colorado
> Boulder, CO 80309

> Cost: $.50

Frostig Developmental Test of Visual Perception (M. Frostig). Palo Alto: Consulting Psychologists Press, 1961.

> The *Frostig Test* measures five operationally defined perceptual skills: eye-motor coordination, figure-ground perception, constancy of shape, position in space, and spatial relationships. This is a paper-and-pencil test designed for young children. Norms are given starting at age four, from which a perceptual quotient may be obtained. There are also a number of worksheet-type, activity-oriented, remedial programs related to test results. Reviewers report the test format to be interesting to young children.

> Available from: Consulting Psychologists Press
> 577 College Avenue
> Palo Alto, CA 94306

> Cost: $ 5.00 Specimen set (test booklet, manual, score key & monograph)
> $ 4.00 Manual & monograph
> $ .75 Score keys
> $ 1.50 Demonstration cards
> $10.00 Examiner's kit (ten test booklets, one manual, one score key, one set of demonstration cards)
> $10.00 pkg. of twenty-five test booklets
> $38.50 pkg. of 100 test booklets

The Functional Profile. Peoria: Peoria Association for Retarded Citizens and United Cerebral Palsy of Peoria, 1974.

> The profile is a checklist of developmental skills to assess children aged birth to six in the social, cognitive, gross motor, fine motor, and self-help areas. The

profile is designed to determine approximate level of developmental functioning and aid in planning an individualized program. The profile may be completed in an hour to an hour-and-a-half by persons who have knowledge and experience with the normal growth and development of infants and young children.

Available from: Constance Smiley
United Cerebral Palsy
913 N. Western Ave.
Peoria, IL 61604

Cost: $.13

Goldman Fristoe Test of Articulation (R. Goldman and M. Fristoe). Circle Pines, MN: American Guidance Service, Inc., 1967.

This test provides a method of assessing an individual's articulation of consonant sounds. There are three subtests. The Sounds-in-Words Subtest utilizes thirty-six pictures of familiar objects; the examiner records the child's articulation of speech sounds. The Sounds-in-Sentences Subtest consists of two stories read aloud by the examiner and illustrated by sets of pictures. In order to approximate speech production of ordinary conversational speech, the child is asked to recount each story in his own words using the pictures as memory aids. The Stimulability Subtest asks the child to pronounce a previously misarticulated phoneme, given both visual and oral stimulation. A filmstrip is available as an alternate method of presenting the *Test*, which the publishers say may be useful for testing immature, easily distracted, or mentally retarded children. The *Test* is designed for children aged two and over, with the results to be recorded on a form which graphically portrays the child's articulatory profile. Percentile rank norms are available for males and females at three-month intervals from age six through sixteen.

Available from: American Guidance Service, Inc.
Publishers Building
Circle Pines, MN 55014

Cost: $22.60 (1320)

Goldman Fristoe Woodcock Test of Auditory Discrimination (R. Goldman, M. Fristoe, and R. Woodcock). Circle Pines, MN: American Guidance Service, Inc., 1970.

This test uses a tape-recorded stimulus and pictures which the child is to select. There are three parts to the instrument: a training procedure, a quiet subtest, and a noise subtest. Each of the two subtests include six words from each of the categories: voiced plosives, unvoiced plosives, voiced continuants, nasals, and unvoiced continuants. The age range is three-years-eight-months through adult. The score consists of the number of errors. Norms are provided for the total test.

Available from: American Guidance Services, Inc.
Publishers Building
Circle Pines, MN 55014

Cost: $23.00 (with cassette) (code 1330)
(reel to reel) (code 1331)

Goodenough Harris Drawing Test (F. Goodenough and D. Harris). Atlanta: The Psychological Corporation, 1963.

This instrument is a nonverbal test of mental ability. The child is asked to draw a man, a woman, and himself. Drawings are scored on the basis of presence or absence of certain characteristics: seventy-three for the man and seventy-one for the woman. There are also Quality Scales which permit a much more rapid estimate of the child's level of maturity when a rough estimate will suffice. Users are cautioned against using this test to make diagnoses of mental impairment, since it is heavily affected by personality variables. It is most useful as a projective tool for clinical assessment. Norms are available for ages three to fifteen, separately for boys and girls, in the form of standard scores and percentile ranks.

Available from: The Psychological Corporation
1372 Peachtree Street, N.E.
Atlanta, GA 30309

Cost: $5.25 (pkg. of thirty-five)
$2.25 Manual
$4.00 Quality scale cards (set of twenty-four)
$6.25 Examiner's kit (manual, quality scale cards, and one test booklet)

Harris Articulation Scale (G. S. Harris). Tucson: University of Arizona, 1973.

The *Harris Articulation Test* was developed for paraprofessionals to use in screening Head Start children. Taking only fifteen minutes to administer, it enables the examiner to identify what sounds a child has trouble producing, and to identify the position (initial, medial, or final) in a word where the child makes his error. The test consists of pictures of objects that stimulate the production of single word responses that have sounds in one of the three positions. Directions are given for materials needed in making and administering the test. This test is available in Spanish.

Available from: Dr. Elizabeth Y. Sharp
Department of Special Education
College of Education
University of Arizona
Tucson, AZ 85721

Cost: $1.25

Houston Test for Language Development. Houston: The Houston Test Company, 1957.

The *Houston Test for Language Development* provides a measure of language development from infancy to the age of six. The *Test* includes two parts. The first part consists of noting characteristics after observation (e.g., "talks to himself spontaneously," "uses present and future," etc.). In the second part, the examiner uses vocabulary cards, miniature objects, crayons, and drawing paper to evaluate the child. The *Test* takes about thirty minutes. Scoring is similar to the *Binet* (normed on a small sample of white children) with basal and ceiling ages for groups of tasks.

Available from: Houston Test Company
                  Post Office Box 35152
                  Houston, TX 77035

Cost: $35.00 + postage for complete kit (0-6)

Illinois Test of Psycholinguistic Ability or ITPA (S. Kirk, J. McCarthy, and W. Kirk). Urbana: University of Illinois Press, 1968.

The ITPA purports to assess twelve aspects of psycholinguistic functioning in children ages two to ten. These twelve aspects, ranging from auditory and visual reception to visual-sequential memory and sound blending, have been conceptualized in terms of three dimensions. First, children's auditory-vocal and visual-motor behaviors comprise abilities labeled "channels of communication." Receptive, organizing, use, and expressive processes comprise the second major dimension, "the psycholinguistic processes." The third dimension consists of two levels instead of processes, "the automatic and the representational." Assessment by way of the ITPA leads to the charting of individual profiles, or underlining intra-individual differences, in terms of these dimensions. Emphasis has been placed upon the identification of major psycholinguistic deficits or disabilities which may require remediation. The ITPA is administered individually. Special training is required for its use.

Available from: University of Illinois Press
                  University of Illinois
                  Urbana, IL 61801

Cost: $58.00

Individual Child Assessment (S. Hering, A. Fazio, and J. Hailey). Piedmont: Circle Preschool, 1975.

The *Individual Child Assessment* was compiled for use by classroom or resource teachers in early childhood programs with children twelve to seventy-two months. It orders skills in six areas of child development: gross motor, fine motor, self-help, social-emotional, cognitive, and language. It assists staff in developmental planning and in individualizing curriculum.

This device helps in charting the child's current functioning, and then in planning to help the child progress to the next level of competence. After assessment, staff members work through a child's strengths to improve the areas of weakness. An accurate and detailed documentation of a child's progress can be obtained by using this instrument over a long period of time.

The instrument was compiled by synthesizing other assessment approaches, by writing the items in behavioral terms, and by including, for the most part, only items that suggest activities appropriate for an early childhood classroom.

Available from: Circle Preschool
                  9 Lake Avenue
                  Piedmont, CA 04611

Cost: $1.50

Infant Evaluation Scale (W. Gingold, P. Gingold, and G. B. Flamer). Fargo, ND: Southeast Mental Health and Retardation Center, 1975

> The *Infant Evaluation Scale* was developed for parents of infants, six weeks to six months, to assess the developmental skill of their child; to share the results with professionals who maintain ongoing cumulative data on the child's development; and to assist the parents in more realistically examining the child's development and the specific activities they can initiate to foster that development. The instrument consists of fifty-three items (not divided into developmental areas) totally administered by the parents of the infant at their leisure. The actual length of time for administration is thirty-five to sixty minutes.

> Available from: Southeast Mental Health and Retardation Center
> 700 First Avenue South
> Fargo, ND 58102

> Cost: $.40

Infant-Parent Training Program Checklist (W. Drezek). Austin: Infant-Parent Training Program, 1973.

> The purpose of the *Checklist* is to assess the developmental level of children functioning between birth and one year of age. The *Checklist*, which has closely spaced behaviors, is divided into five main developmental areas: cognition (three subareas), communication (three subareas), social, gross motor, and self-help. The *Checklist* will take a teacher one to two hours to administer. When the *Checklist* is completed, the teacher should have found the functioning level of the child in each of the five areas. The teacher can use the scale in two ways to assist in programming: in building individual activities and in progress evaluation. A testing manual and curriculum is available.

> Available from: Infant-Parent Training Program
> 1226 East 9th Street
> Austin, TX 78701

> Cost: $.90

Informal Teacher Assessment Instrument (W. Drezek). Austin: Infant-Parent Training Program, 1975.

> The purpose of the *Informal Teacher Assessment Instrument* is to determine the approximate developmental level of a child, to sample a range of the child's behavior in a natural setting, and to attune the teacher to specific qualitative aspects of behavior in all areas of development. The instrument can be used: (1) as a teaching device to train teachers in assessment, (2) for progress in evaluation, and (3) for program development.

> The instrument incorporates developmental checklists, skill checklists, questions, and observation guidelines to produce an assessment of children, zero to six years of age. The instrument can be used in a classroom setting by the teacher or in an individual testing situation. Administration time is one to two hours.

A paper on using the instrument and applications for planning, along with planning forms, are also available.

Available from: Wendy Drezek
 Infant-Parent Training Program
 1226 East 9th Street
 Austin, TX 78701

Cost: $1.00

Kindergarten Evaluation of Learning Potential or KELP (J. A. R. Wilson, M. C. Robeck). Manchester: McGraw-Hill, Webster Division, 1967.

This instrument predicts school success in the early grades based on the learning that a child actually does in kindergarten. It is designed as both a teaching and evaluation instrument. KELP items include skipping, color identification, bead design, bolt board, block design, calendar, number boards, safety signs, writing a name, auditory perception, and social interaction. The latter nine items are rated at three levels: association, concept formation, and creative self-expression. The items are taught by the teacher, who observes and records the accomplishment of the tasks over the entire kindergarten year. Classroom materials, teaching tips, and a summary retention test are available. The authors report that stanine norms can be obtained on request. The results of a survey of the views of teachers, who have used KELP, on the topics of construct validity, correlations with *Stanford-Binet*, and predictive validities with teacher ratings (first grade) and *Metropolitan Achievement Test* scores are available. No reliability studies are reported.

Available from: Webster Division
 McGraw-Hill Book Company
 Manchester Road
 Manchester, MO 63011

Cost: $164.52 (complete kit)

Koontz Child Developmental Program: Training Activities for the First 48 Months (C. Koontz). Los Angeles: Western Psychological Services, 1974.

The *Koontz Child Developmental Program* is intended for use by teachers, parents, psychologists, therapists, and pediatricians with children who function between the ages of one and forty-eight months. This instrument was designed to give adults working with children a tool to assess the child's functioning level in gross motor, fine motor, social, and language skills. Performance items were selected from existing scales with the following criteria: (1) they must be observable; (2) they must be able to be described; (3) they must be developmental; and (4) they must allow the adult to observe and record the successful accomplishment of the performance item in an informal manner. Items are arranged by age levels in twenty-two increments with a total of 550 performance items. Training activities, included for each performance item, are suggested for use in planning a program for the child. The assessment of a child is recorded on the Record Card which is divided into developmental areas and months.

Available from: Western Psychological Services
12031 Wilshire Boulevard
Los Angeles, CA 90025

Cost: $12.00 Kit
$ 4.50 Record card (1 pkg. of twenty-five)
$ 3.25 Record card (2-19 pkgs. of twenty-five)
$ 2.75 Record card (20 or more pkgs. of twenty-five)

Learning Accomplishment Profile (A. Sanford). Winston-Salem, N.C.: Kaplan School Supply, 1975.

The *Learning Accomplishment Profile* is designed to provide the teacher of handicapped preschool children with a simple, behavior-oriented evaluation of the child's skills. For the first section, tasks were taken from many developmental scales and are arranged hierarchically, with developmental ages from the scale from which the item was taken indicated. Areas covered are: gross motor, fine motor, social skills, self-help, cognitive, and language development. For each task there is a column in which to indicate the entry test date, the date the test was achieved, and comments. The *Profile*'s second section is geared more to specific instructional objectives. The teacher can indicate attainment of specific criterion levels for numerous skills in the areas of writing, self-help, and cognitive development (including communication skills). No procedure for obtaining scores is given, but one could get a rough developmental age from the items completed in the first section.

Available from: Kaplan School Supply
600 Jonestown Road
Winston-Salem, NC 27103

Cost: $ 2.00 Learning accomplishment profile
$ 2.50 Manual
$150.00 Diagnostic edition assessment kit
$ 3.00 Infant learning accomplishment profile

Learning Accomplishment Profile-Diagnostic Edition (P. M. Griffen, A. R. Sanford, and D. C. Wilson). Winston Salem, NC: Kaplan School Supply, 1975

The purpose of the *Learning Accomplishment Profile-Diagnostic Edition* (LAP-D) is to provide a standardized, criterion-referenced instrument for assessment. This instrument is based on the prescriptive LAP which is an assessment instrument from which educational objectives can be derived and prescriptive programs can be established.

Applicable to ages ranging from twelve months to six years, teachers or trained paraprofessionals can administer the instrument in three-fourths of an hour to two hours. However, the examiner must adhere to the rigidly specified procedures and criteria contained in the manual.

The LAP-D is divided into five skill areas: gross motor, fine motor, self-help, cognitive, and language. Each of these general skill areas is further broken down into subskills. Within these subskills, tasks are sequenced from least to most difficult. It is easy to administer and score.

Standardization and validity studies are in process.

The complete set includes the Examiner's Manual, score sheets, and kit materials (durable, reusable · materials: attractive original pictures and puzzles with brightly colored objects).

Available from: Kaplan School Supply Corporation
600 Jonestown Road
Winston Salem, NC 27103

Cost: $150.00

Learning Accomplishment Profile for Infants: Experimental Edition (P. M. Griffen and A. R. Sanford). Winston-Salem, NC: Kaplan School Supply Corporation, 1975.

The *Learning Accomplishment Profile for Infants* (LAP-I) is designed to provide the parent or teacher of the handicapped infant, aged zero to three, with a simple criterion-referenced record of the child's existing skills. The LAP-I identifies the next appropriate step in the development of the individual child and gives detailed instructions for reaching this objective. Short directions and recording space are also provided in convenient chart form. There is no set amount of time for administering the LAP-I. The child is observed during normal daily activities.

The LAP-I is a sixty-four-page book in loose-leaf format, perforated and punched for a ring binder. It is divided into two sections.

Section I - Developmental Data. A hierarchy of behavior listed in developmental sequence and drawn from the most recent normative data provides the basis of an evaluation of the infant's existing skills in six areas of development: gross motor, fine motor, social, self help, cognitive, and language.

Section II - Instructional Units. Detailed instructions and recording charts provide a method for the teaching of important behaviors in the sequence of development.

Available from: Kaplan School Supply Corporation
600 Jonestown Road
Winston-Salem, NC 27103

Cost: $3.00

The Lexington Developmental Scale (J. Irwin, C. A. Coleman, et al.). Lexington: Child Development Centers, Inc., 1974.

The Lexington Developmental Scale (LDS) was designed to be used by the teacher as an instrument for assessing children, as an aid in helping parents to understand their child better, as a basis for curriculum planning for the total class and especially for the individual child, and as a means of evaluating the progress of the individual child as well as a means for evaluating the class program.

The scale evaluates five important areas in the development of the child: motor, language, personal and social, cognitive, and emotional. Each of the first four areas is scored on the basis of developmental age. The fifth area, emotional, is scored on a five-point scale because there are inadequate age norms in this area.

The LDS is available in two age ranges: for the infant, which is appropriate for children in the birth to two years age range; and for early childhood, which is appropriate for children in the two to six years age range. Using test-retest techniques, both scales have yielded high coefficients of correlations.

Validity has been assumed for both of the full scales because: (1) the age placement of the individual test items is based on a detailed search of the literature; (2) the progression of items within each sequence reflects the judgment of experienced teachers and clinicians; and (3) the chronological ages and developmental ages of children tested have shown substantial agreement both by item and by areas.

In the full LDS there are 452 items. The shortened version of the LDS was developed primarily for clinic and home use where there is limited time, space, and equipment. It is possible for the scale to be administered in a time period of thirty minutes.

Available from: The Child Development Centers of U.C.P.B.
Post Office Box 8003
465 Springhill Drive
Lexington, KY 40503

Cost: $5.00 LDS manual
$1.50 LDS screening form manual
$ .30 Charts
$4.00 Innovative instructional materials book

Marshalltown Behavioral Development Profile (M. Donahue, J. Montgomery, and others). Marshalltown, IA: AEA #6 Preschool Division, 1975.

This *Profile* was developed for handicapped and culturally deprived children in the zero to six year range. It is designed to facilitate individualized prescriptive teaching of preschool children within the home setting. Items are based upon normal development and are taken from other standardized scales. The *Profile* contains a list of 327 developmental skills collapsed into three general categories: communication, motor, and social. The items within each category are arranged according to age. The device is criterion-referenced and is designed to measure the progress of each child in months.

The *Profile* is used with a score sheet and in conjunction with the Behavioral Prescription Guides (Manuals IIa, IIb, and IIc). The guides list behavioral objectives and the activities to accomplish each objective. There are objectives for each of the skills measured in the *Profile*.

The results from the *Profile* are used to ascertain the child's level of development as well as his strengths and weaknesses. The person who is working with the child then uses this information to set objectives and choose strategies for accomplishing those objectives.

Available from: AEA #6, Preschool Division
507 East Anson
Marshalltown, IA 50158

Cost: $3.00

McCarthy Scales of Children's Abilities (D. McCarthy). New York: The Psychological Corporation, 1972

The *McCarthy Scales of Children's Abilities* (MSCA) was developed to satisfy the need for a single instrument to determine general intellectual level as well as strengths and weaknesses of children two-and-a-half through eight-and-a-half years of age. The MSCA is composed of eighteen separate tests which have been grouped into six scales: verbal, perceptual-performance, quantitative, general cognitive, memory, and motor. Administration time is approximately forty-five minutes for children under five and approximately an hour for older children. For each of the six scales, the child's raw score is converted to a scaled score called an index. Fifteen of the eighteen tests are cognitive and compose the General Cognitive Scale. The General Cognitive Index describes the child's functioning at a given point in time and should be viewed in the context of his Indexes on the other five scales. It is the child's profile of scores rather than one particular score that indicates his developmental maturity, strengths, and weaknesses. The MSCA was standardized on a stratified sample of 1032 cases, and on an average of 100 children per six-month interval from two-and-a-half to five-and-a-half and on a per year interval from five-and-a-half to eight-and-a-half. The technical information available indicates good reliability and validity data available.

Available from: Psychological Corporation
304 E. 45th Street
New York, NY 10017

Cost: $59.00 Set with manual (6D019)

Meeting Street School Screening Test in *Early Identification of Children with Learning Disabilities: The Meeting Street Providence* (P. Hainsworth and E. M. Siqueland). East Providence, RI: Crippled Children and Adults of Rhode Island Incorporated, 1969.

The *Meeting Street School Screening Test* (MSSST) is an individually administered screening test for children between five and seven-and-a-half years of age. The twenty-minute test is designed to screen children in the motor, visual perceptual, and language areas. The instrument may be administered by trained teachers, nonprofessionals, psychologists, and/or physicians. Norms are provided at half-year intervals. The instrument was standardized on 500 kindergarten and first grade children who were selected to represent the population, socio-economically, on the basis of 1966 U.S. census figures. It was normed on the scores of 100 children per each half-year. Reliability and validity have been established.

Available from: Meeting Street School
667 Waterman Avenue
East Providence, RI 02914

Cost: $12.00 Manual
$ 5.00 for 50 record forms
$ 9.00 for 100 record forms

Memphis Comprehensive Development Scales (A. P. Quick, T. L. Little, A. A. Campbell). Belmont: Fearon Publishers, 1974.

The *Comprehensive Developmental Scale* is designed to determine a child's level of functioning in five areas: personal-social, gross motor, fine motor, language skills, and perceptual-cognitive. This is an instrument for assessing development at levels which can be used in planning individualized-prescriptive-educational programs for preschool developmentally delayed children.

The scale is composed of five subscales representing the five areas of development. There are 260 skill items listed on the five subscales. These items are arranged in sequential order and in three-month intervals from zero to five years.

The set of materials includes the Developmental Skills Assignment Record, a sheet for assigning individual skills, and the Continuous Record for Educational-Development Gain for recording and evaluating the child's mastery of skills, both qualitatively and quantitatively. In addition, there is a Guide to Programming which tells how to use the three forms.

Any person with training in and knowledge of preschool development can administer the instrument.

Available from: Fearon Publishers
6 Davis Drive
Belmont, CA 94002

Costs: $ 1.50 for one set
$11.00 for twenty-five sets

Metropolitan Readiness Tests (G. Hildreth, N. Griffiths, and M. McGauvran). Atlanta: The Psychological Corporation, 1976.

Six subtests comprise the *Metropolitan* battery: work meaning, listening comprehension, perceptual recognition of similarities, recognition of lowercase alphabet letters, number knowledge, and perceptual-motor control (copying). In combination, these tests are intended to provide an assessment of children's development in skills that contribute to "readiness for first grade instruction." The *Metropolitan* battery is ordinarily given at the end of kindergarten or the beginning of first grade. Results may be used to classify pupils on a "readiness" continuum. Such a classification is presumed to be helpful for teachers who desire more efficient management of their instructional efforts. At least minimal skill in the use of writing instruments and paper is prerequisite for children to whom the *Metropolitan* is administered. However, no special training is needed by teachers for the administration and scoring of these tests. Norms are based upon a nationwide sample of beginning first graders. In general, the reliability of these tests is high and their predictive validity is encouraging. The *Metropolitan* is among the most popular batteries currently used in public school kindergartens and primary grades.

Available from: The Psychological Corporation
1372 Peachtree Street, N.E.
Atlanta, GA 30309

Cost: $11.75 (pkg. of thirty-five)
Level I & II (Kindergarten and 1st grade)

Milani-Comparetti Motor Developmental Test (P. Pearson, L. Rice, J. Trembath). Omaha: Meyer Children's Rehabilitation Institute, 1973.

The *Milani-Comparetti Motor Developmental Test* is a simple, rapid, standardized-neurodevelopmental screening examination designed to evaluate a child's physical development from birth to about two years. The Meyer Children's Rehabilitation Institute (MCRI) staff has modified the original chart by A. Milani-Comparetti and E. A. Gidoni and developed *A Manual of the Milani-Comparetti Testing Procedures* to teach the correct procedures. The original is divided into two sections, i.e., an upper "behavioristic scale" and a lower section for the primitive and/or evoked reactions. The MCRI modification simply puts the items in the order in which they are generally administered.

A physician, therapist, or public health nurse can determine, within five to ten minutes, whether one child's physical development corresponds to that of a normal child's. Administered several times over a period of months, the test indicates trends in a child's motor development. This information can be used to detect such problems as cerebral palsy, motor delay, asymmetry, and mental deficiency.

Available from: Meyer Children's Rehabilitation Institute
University of Nebraska Medical Center
Omaha, NB 69131

Cost: $1.75

Minnesota Preschool Scale (F. Goodenough and others). Circle Pines, MN: American Guidance Service, Inc., 1940.

This scale is used to assess development of mental ability in children of ages six months to five years. Two parallel forms are available. Items pertain to pointing out parts of the body or objects; naming familiar objects; copying; imitative drawing; block building; response to pictures; Knox cube imitation; obeying simple commands; comprehension; discrimination, recognition, or tracing of forms; naming objects from memory; colors; incomplete pictures; picture puzzles; digit spans; paper folding; absurdities; vocabulary; imitating clock hands; and speech. The test has verbal, nonverbal, and total scores for children three to five years of age, and total scores for younger children. The instrument is individually administered and paced. The examiner should have considerable experience in the testing of young children and some practice with the test materials. Age C scores and percent placement norms and I.Q. equivalents are not available. Inter-form reliabilities, but no other technical data, are reported.

Available from: American Guidance Service, Inc.
Publishers Building
Circle Pines, MN 55014

Cost: $43.00 Complete kit (code 1240)

Missouri Children's Picture Series (J. Sines, J. Pauker, and L. Sines). Iowa City: Psychological Assessment and Services, 1972.

The *Missouri Children's Picture Series* is a personality test which can be administered to children of varying ages and abilities. It consists of 238 simple line drawings, each on a numbered 3 x 5 card. The pictures show a child engaged in a variety of activities and situations. The child is asked to decide whether each picture looks like something he would like to do. The child puts the cards that look like fun to him on one pile, the others on another. The examiner retrieves the piles and later sorts and scores the pictures. The manual says most children complete the test in fifteen minutes by themselves. It can be administered to nonverbal or physically handicapped children. Scoring aids are provided for the eight scales: conformity, masculinity-femininity, maturity, aggression, inhibition, activity level, sleep disturbance, and somatization. Standard score distributions, derived from test results of 3,877 children, are given as "T" score equivalents, separately for males and females for each year from age five to sixteen.

Available from: Psychological Assessment and Services
P.O. Box 1031
Iowa City, IA 52240

Cost: $25.00 Specimen set

Move-Grow-Learn Survey (R. E. Orpet and L. L. Huestis). Chicago: Follett Publishing Company, 1967.

This survey was developed to assist classroom teachers, movement education supervisors, school psychologists, and other professional school personnel in evaluating selected aspects of a child's motor development. It is intended for use with Frostig and Maslows' *Move-Grow-Learn* curriculum and with *Movement Education: Theory and Practice.*

Eight broad areas of sensory-motor and movement skills are included: coordination and rhythm, balance, flexibility, strength, speed, endurance (only children eight years old or older should be rated on endurance), and body awareness. For each subarea, illustrative activities and room for comments are included.

This is not a standardized, psychometric instrument in which developmental norms are provided for each age level. The assessment is based upon the examiner's observations of the child in classroom, playground, and gymnasium activities.

Ratings are from one through five: one=severely impaired; two=mildly impaired; three=adequate; four=good; and five=excellent.

Children rated one or two need considerable training in the skill or skills in which they are deficient. Children rated three should have training; and children rated four and five can also benefit from movement education.

Move-Grow-Learn activities are suggested for additional training in skills in which a child is rated one, two, or three.

Available from: Follett Publishing Co.
1010 W. Washington Blvd.
Chicago, IL 60607

Cost: $12.96 Program (3530)
$ 2.10 Specimen set (3534)

Northwestern Syntax Screening Test (L. Lee). Evanston: Northwestern University Press, 1971.

This test was designed as a structured screening test for deficits in both expressive and receptive use of syntax for children three through eight years of age.

The test consists of a series of pictures. The procedure is structured for both the comprehension and production portions. It takes approximately twenty minutes to administer and does not require a great deal of experience.

Norms are based upon 242 children between three and eleven years. There is no published reliability data.

Available from: Northwestern University Press
1735 Benson Avenue
Evanston, IL 60201

Cost: $10.00

Oseretsky Test of Motor Proficiency (E. A. Doll, ed.). Circle Pines, MN: American Guidance Service, Inc., 1946.

The *Oseretsky Test of Motor Proficiency* is an adaptation of a very old test developed in Russia. In the present form, there are six tasks given for each age (whole years from four to sixteen). The tasks sample general static coordination, motor-speed, simultaneous voluntary movements, and performance without extraneous movements. The Test requires twenty to thirty minutes to administer. In its use of age level tasks, it is similar to the *Binet*. Instructions are given in calculating the motor age.

Available from: American Guidance Service, Inc.
Publishers Building
Circle Pines, MN 55014

Cost: $35.00 Complete set (1280)

Peabody Individual Achievement Test (L. M. Dunn and F. Markwardt). Circle Pines, MN: American Guidance Service, Inc., 1970.

The *Peabody Individual Achievement Test* is an individually administered, achievement-screening test in mathematics, reading, spelling, and general information. It requires thirty to forty minutes and uses conventional basal-ceiling procedures. It yields six scores: mathematics, reading recognition, reading comprehension, spelling, general information, and total. Norms are given for ages five and up as grade equivalents, age equivalents, percentile ranks by age or grade, and standard scores by age or grade. The test requires no writing—only oral or pointing responses.

Available from: American Guidance Service, Inc.
Publishers Building
Circle Pines, MN 55014

Costs: $32.00 Regular edition (1410)
$41.00 Special edition (1411)

Peabody Picture Vocabulary Test or PPVT (L. M. Dunn). Circle Pines, MN: American Guidance Service, Inc., 1965.

The PPVT is assumed to measure recognition (hearing) vocabulary by having a child identify correct pictorial representations (from among four alternatives) in a series as the examiner speaks a word corresponding to each picture. It was originally designed to predict school success, and results obtained from its use are often taken as rough estimates of a child's "verbal intelligence." Items are arranged from simple to complex. This test is suitable for use with children of preschool age and beyond and is easily administered. Further, the PPVT requires little in the way of special training for scoring and interpretation. In general, reliability of the test is satisfactory, and scores derived from its use are correlated positively with a wide range of other measures of verbal behavior. Of studies performed to date relevant to the validity of the PPVT for predicting school success, it appears that the test is more effective with children beyond age seven than with those of nursery and kindergarten age. Extensive use has been made of the PPVT for the study of mentally retarded children.

Available from: American Guidance Service, Inc.
Publishers Building
Circle Pines, MN 55014

Cost: $14.00 Regular (1110)
$19.50 Special (1111)

The Perceptual Skills Curriculum (J. Rosner). New York: Walker and Co., 1973

The four programs of this curriculum can be used by teachers either concurrently or consecutively, depending on need, with classes of K-2 children developmentally and K-6 remedially. Each program is organized around a sequence of behavioral objectives which children master successively by completing the correlated tests and learning activities found in each program. A pretest/post test pattern is used to measure progress.

The instructor may use all four programs or concentrate on any one, with individuals, small groups, or classes of twenty-five to thirty children. Pupil Profile Progress Charts are included in each program. The programs are: I, Visual-Motor Skills; II, Auditory-Motor Skills; III, General-Motor Skills; and IV, Introducing Letters and Numerals.

Available from: Walker Educational Book Corporation
720 Fifth Avenue
New York, NY 10019

Cost: $66.00 Complete set (school price)
$ 5.50 Introductory Guide

$18.70 Visual-Motor Skills
$11.50 Auditory-Motor Skills
$ 6.60 General-Motor Skills
$32.50 Introducing Letters and Numerals (two volumes)

Portage Guide to Early Education, revised edition (S. Bluma, M. Shearer, A. Frohman, and J. Hilliard). Portage: Portage Project, 1976.

The *Portage Guide to Early Education* is comprised of three parts: a checklist, a manual, and cards to be used in teaching behaviors included in the checklist. The checklist is to be used as an assessment tool to pinpoint existing skills in the child's behavioral repertoire, as well as behavior the child has yet to learn. The checklist also provides a method of maintaining an ongoing record of a child's progress. The instrument was developed to assess children between the ages of birth and six in six areas of development, including infant stimulation. There are 580 developmentally sequenced behaviors.

Available from: Portage Project
412 East Slifer Street
Portage, WI 53901

Cost: $32.00 + postage for set of materials (includes fifteen checklists, cards and manual)
$ 6.50 + postage for packet of fifteen checklists

Preschool Attainment Record (E. A. Doll). Circle Pines, MN: American Guidance Service, INC., 1966.

The instrument combines an assessment of physical, social, and intellectual functions in a global appraisal of children from birth to seven years of age. The *Record* includes eight categories of developmental behavior: ambulation, manipulation, rapport, communication, responsibility, information, ideation, and creativity. For each category, there is one item for each six-month age span. The item types, item arrangement, testing procedures, and interviewer qualifications are the same as for the *Vineland Social Maturity Scale* described later. Mean age for expected performance of each behavior is provided. Total scores may be converted to attainment ages or attainment quotients. No reliability or validity studies are yet available.

Available from: American Guidance Service, Inc.
Publishers Building
Circle Pines, MN 55014

Cost: $2.90 Package of twenty-five (1181)
$1.60 Manual (1182)

Preschool Inventory, revised edition (B. Caldwell). Reading, MA: Addison-Wesley, 1970.

This instrument was designed in relation to Project Head Start. Its purpose is to assess achievement in areas regarded as necessary foundations for early school success. These areas have been labeled concept-activation-sensory, concept-activation-numerical, personal-social responsiveness, and associative vocabulary. The *Preschool Inventory* has been used as a rough diagnostic test; that is, it has been used to identify selected "cultural handicaps" and as a gross measure of the impact of Head Start experience on children. Limited norms are provided (based on the performance of children, ages two to six-and-a-half, identified as products of "lower" and "middle-class" backgrounds). Like so many preschool tests, this inventory must also be administered individually. The reliability of this test appears to meet acceptable standards, although no empirical statement of validity is reported in the test manual.

Available from: Addison-Wesley Publishing Company
Reading, MA 01967

Cost: $2.75 (English) Pkg. of twenty
$3.00 (Spanish) Pkg. of twenty
$3.00 Specimen set
$2.00 Handbook (English and Spanish)

Preschool Language Scale (I. L. Zimmerman, U. G. Steiner, and R. L. Fvatt). Columbus: Charles E. Merrill Publishing Company, 1969.

The *Scale* is designed to detect language strengths and deficiencies. It consists of two main parts—Auditory Comprehension and Verbal Ability—and includes a supplementary Articulation Section. The test is designed for ages one to eight. Developmental ages are given for items. From these ages, an auditory comprehension quotient and a verbal ability quotient can be derived, as well as a general language quotient. Reviewers caution against relying heavily on such scores, although developmental ages can be useful for screening. The *Scale* is considered to be a sophisticated, informal inventory.

Available from: Charles E. Merrill Publishing Company
1300 Alum Creek Drive
Columbus, OH 43216

Cost: $8.95 Manual, sample scale, picture book
$6.95 Pkg. of scales - ten per pkg.

Preschool Screening System: Start of a Longitudinal Preventive Approach, Field Test Edition, 1974 (P. Hainsworth and M. Hainsworth). Pawtucket: First Step Publications, 1974.

The *Preschool Screening System* (PSS) consists of a child test and a parent questionnaire for children three to five-years-and-four-months. The PSS is an individually administered screening test, fifteen to twenty-five minutes in length. The PSS screens information processing skills in language, visual motor, and gross motor skills. The parent questionnaire, fifteen to twenty-five minutes in length, includes items regarding behavioral characteristics of the child's skills and "behavior at home" as well as a short medical and developmental history. Scores and totals can be converted into eight percentile ranges through tables of norms provided at four-month intervals. The PSS can be administered by an experienced examiner or trained technician, or by a volunteer, or a paraprofessional supervised by an experienced examiner. The manual contains sections called an "Overview of the Preschool Screening System, Implementing an Early Screening Program" and "Using the Results." It also contains administration and scoring directions. The PSS uses the same theoretical model and format as the *Meeting Street School Screening Test*. Normative data for the field test edition were obtained from over 600 children during a two-year period. Reliability and validity information are adequate. Further technical data will be gathered in the development of the final version.

Available from: First Step Publications
Box 1635
Pawtucket, RI 02862

Cost: $ 7.50 Manual
$ 6.00 100 Test forms
$10.00 100 Parent questionnaires

Primary Mental Abilities (T. G. Thurstone). Chicago: Science Research Associates, Inc., 1963.

These tests are designed to provide both multifactored and general measures of intelligence. The five "primary mental abilities" measured by the tests are verbal meaning (understanding of ideas expressed in words), number facility, reasoning, perceptual speed, and spatial relations. The test requires a little over an hour and may be given to small groups. It is usually given in two sessions. The perceptual speed test requires timing. The test is given from a test booklet; no additional materials are required. Mental age equivalents for each part and for the total test are given. The test is designed for pupils in kindergarten and first grade.

Available from: Science Research Associates, Inc.
259 East Erie Street
Chicago, IL 60611

Cost: $7.20 package of twenty-five

The Psychiatric Behavior Scale (W. F. Barker, L. Sandler, A. Borneman, G. Knight, F. Humphrys, S. Risan). Philadelphia: The Franklin Institute Research Laboratories, 1973.

The *Psychiatric Behavior Rating Scale* (PBS) assesses a preschool child's emotional development. The scale can be used with children two-and-a-half to six-and-a-half years old. The subscales assess expression of aggression, relationships, independence-dependence, impulse control, reaction to stress; need for communication; appropriate coordination, appropriate feeling; and bizarre behaviors. The instrument takes five to seven minutes to administer and should be administered by a teacher or day-care worker who has had at least one month's contact with the child.

The PBS was developed as an instrument to assess longitudinally the emotional development of preschool children with problems. The instrument can be used as a guide for the day-care worker to identify specific areas of development which may need remediation, as well as for screening. Technical data regarding standardization, reliability, and validity are available from the developers.

Available from: Louise Sandler
Center for Preschool Services
The Franklin Institute Research Laboratories
20th and Race Streets
Philadelphia, PA 19103

Cost: $ .20

Pupil Progress Evaluation Plan (J. Dickerson, M. Evanson, and L. Spurlock). Coeur d'Alene, ID: Panhandle Child Development Association Inc., 1975.

The *Pupil Progress Evaluation Plan* was designed: (1) to give early childhood educators a concise, useful, time-saving way to administer a basic pre- and postdevelopmental assessment; (2) to help in arriving at long term objectives for children; (3) to help in recording cumulative skills accomplished; and (4) to assist in recording time sampled data (when appropriate) so that ongoing individual pupil progress information will be readily available for teachers and parents who wish to assess the program's effectiveness.

Teachers or trained aides of children, zero to six, can record assessment and individual pupil progress information over a yearly period. Each form includes two carbon copies so the teacher may return data to the administrator or parents and still have a copy for records.

The instrument includes a developmental assessment, a pupil objective program schedule, a cumulative task accomplishment sheet, observation recording forms, and a pupil progress graph. Instructions are included for each form.

Available from: Panhandle Child Development Association, Inc.
421 1/2 Sherman Avenue
Coeur d'Alene, ID 83814

Cost: $1.50 per copy plus postage and handling

Referral Form Checklist of Problem Behaviors (RFCL) in *The Rutland Center Model for Treating Emotionally Disturbed Children* (M. M. Wood). Athens: Rutland Center, 1975.

The RFCL may be used both as an assessment instrument and as a pre-post-measure to document a child's (age three to fourteen years) problems and the severity of those problems as perceived by the parents, teachers, and professional staff or the special placement program. Part I, fifty-four behavior problems, is organized into four major developmental areas: behavior, communication, socialization, and academic or pre-academic skills. Each problem is rated on a scale from one, "high priority problem," to five, "not a problem or not noticed." Only Part I is used with parents and classroom teachers. Part II is composed of diagnostic classification, and a view of the problem including a rating of severity and prognosis which the professional staff must complete. Length of time for administration ranges from twenty minutes to one hour.

The instrument with directions, supplementary sections, and summary procedures are contained in *The Rutland Center Model for Treating Emotionally Disturbed Children*.

Available from: The Technical Assistance Office
698 North Pope Street
Athens, GA 30601

Cost: $5.00

Scales of Early Communication Skills for Hearing-Impaired Children (J. S. Moog, A. V. Geers). St. Louis: Central Institute for the Deaf, 1975.

The *Scales of Early Communication Skills for Hearing-Impaired Children* is designed to assess speech and language development of hearing-impaired children between the ages of two and eight years. The scales are designed to be given by the teacher. The information obtained through the use of the scales is the first step in establishing realistic teaching objectives. The instrument includes four scales: receptive language, expressive language, nonverbal receptive, and nonverbal expressive.

Each scale contains a large number of levels which represent steps in the acquisition of skills which can be used as guidelines for teaching. Each item includes a rationale, criteria for rating the skill, and the demonstration of the skill to enable the teacher to describe precisely the behaviors which demonstrate the child's ability to perform at that level. The scales were standardized on 372 deaf children between two-year-zero-months and eight-years-eleven-months. Other technical data indicate a moderate to high degree of inter-rater reliability.

Available from: Central Institute for the Deaf
818 South Euclid Avenue
St. Louis, MO 63110

Cost: $ 7.50 Manual and one scale (C10 301)
$ 3.00 Twenty-five scales to a package
$10.00 Introductory set - one manual and twenty-five scales

School Readiness Survey or SRS (F. L. Jordan and J. Massey). Palo Alto: Consulting Psychologists Press, 1967.

The instrument is designed to help the parent understand the capacities and developmental needs of his child, aged four to six. The items require the child to choose an appropriate picture, figure, word, or symbol, or to answer orally. Subscores are: number concepts, discrimination of form, color naming, symbol matching, speaking vocabulary, listening vocabulary, and general information. SRS is parent administered and paced. The total score and each subscore are related to likelihood of readiness. Suggestions as to how the parent can aid his child, in each area, to be ready for school are included. Cumulative percentage norms for total score and each subscore by sex are available. Test-retest (June/October) reliabilities and correlations of SRS scores with kindergarten teachers' ratings are reported.

Available from: Consulting Psychologists Press
577 College Ave.
Palo Alto, CA 94306

Cost: $ 1.00 Specimen set (manual & test)
     $ .75 Manual
     $ 12.50 Test booklets - package of 25
     $ 47.00   "   "   "   100
     $120.00   "   "   "   500

Search and Teach (A. Silver and R. Hagin). New York: Walker and Co., 1977.

This program detects learning difficulties in five- and six-year-old children and helps prevent later school failure. *Search* is an individual test, designed to be given to all children in a class during the kindergarten year or in the early months of first grade. Administration and scoring of the test takes approximately twenty minutes. It consists of ten component subtests: three tests of visual perception (matching, recall, and visual-motor), two auditory tests (discrimination and sequencing), two intermodal tests (articulation and initial consonants), and three body image tests (directionality, finger schema, and pencil grip).

Teach is a resource book of instructional material designed to prevent learning failure by teaching the skills the vulnerable child needs for steady progress in reading, writing, and spelling. First, each child's specific deficits are delineated by *Search*; next, the teacher selects from the sequenced activities in *Teach* those that will meet the child's specific needs. Typically, *Teach* is used on a one-to-one basis (or in small groups) in a resource room, the corner of a classroom, or clinic. The activities can be taught by a classroom teacher, a resource room teacher or an educational assistant. The learning tasks of *Teach* are sequenced within clusters of perceptual skills to mesh with the components of *Search.*

Available from: Walker Educational Book Corporation
                720 Fifth Ave.
                New York, NY 10019

Costs: $24.00 *Search* Kit (includes following three items)
     $ 9.50 *Search* Manual
     $ 6.00 *Search* Record Blanks (Set of 30)
     $ 9.00 *Search* Identification Toys
     $36.50 *Teach*

SEEC Developmental Wheel (J. E. Swanson and Staff). Schaumburg: Early Childhood Education, 1976

The *SEEC Developmental Wheel* may be used for screening, diagnosis, educational planning, parent reporting, and program evaluation. It can also be used for teacher and parent training in child development.

Professionals, parents, aides, or other personnel trained in its administration can use the wheel to assess the behaviors of children, birth through five, in five areas of development.

The "mini-wheel" specifies twelve developmental milestones (with criteria for mastery) in five areas of development: intellectual (based upon Piaget), social-emotional, self-help, motor, and language. The "maxi-wheel" provides an extensive developmental sequence in the five areas for purposes of assessment and educational planning.

Available from: Jennie E. Swanson
Early Childhood Education
804 West Bode Road
Schaumburg, IL 60194

Cost: $5.00 Sample packet (mini-wheel, maxi-wheel, and instructions)

SEED Developmental Profiles (J. Herst, S. Wolfe, E. Jorgensen, and S. Pallam). Denver: Sewall Early Education Developmental Program, 1975.

The *SEED Developmental Profiles* were developed in order to obtain a functional assessment of severely handicapped children's development from birth through forty-eight months. The SEED scales assess a child in seven developmental areas including social-emotional, gross motor, fine motor, adaptive reasoning, speech and language, feeding, dressing, and simple hygiene. Items from standardized instruments were selected for the profiles. The profiles can be used by professionals or paraprofessionals who have experience in working with young, severely handicapped children. The profiles were designed to provide a framework for developing individual goals and objectives for a child. There is a profile for each developmental area as well as a master profile for summary data for each of the seven developmental areas. Items for the first year are given in four-week increments and then in increments of three months until the child reaches forty-eight months.

Available from: SEED Program
Sewall Rehabilitation Center
1360 Vine
Denver, CO 80206

Cost: $2.25

SEED Reflex and Therapeutic Evaluation (G. Jorgenson, S. Wolfe, and P. Pollan). Denver: Sewall Rehabilitation Center, 1975.

The purpose of the *SEED Reflex and Therapeutic Evaluation* is: (1) to obtain a clinical picture of oral and body reflex development, breathing, posturing, muscle tone, general muscle strength, joint range of motion, sensation and skin condition; and (2) to obtain an oral peripheral examination.

Section I lists nine oral reflexes and the appropriate times for their emergence and assimilation. Section II lists thirty-six body reflexes, divided into categories called movement reflexes of newborn, brain stimulation level, midbrain level, equilibrium reactions, and additional movement reflexes and responses. Section III is an oral peripheral examination including facial symmetry; dentition, tongue, lip, palate, and jaw mobility and control; and an assessment format of diadochokinesis and breath support. Section IV has space for commenting on breathing, posturing, muscle tone, muscle strength, range of motion sensation, skin condition, and hand preference.

In one hour two persons such as physical and/or occupational therapists, speech and language pathologists, or anyone with a working knowledge of reflex development and/or oral structure can administer the evaluation. It can be used with target populations ranging in age from birth through life.

Available from: SEED Program
Sewall Rehabilitation Center
1360 Vine
Denver, CO 80206

Cost: $ .15

The Slosson Intelligence Test (R. L. Slosson). Los Angeles: Western Psychological Services, 1963.

> *The Slosson Intelligence Test* (SIT) is a simple individual screening instrument consisting of vocabulary, memory, reasoning, and motor items for children birth through adulthood. The technical data in the manual state, "The validity of the I.Q.'s obtained on infants and children under four years according to much of the research is unsatisfactory." The validity and reliability data for children under four are minimal. However, for individuals aged four through adulthood there is adequate reliability and validity data. This instrument is similar in nature to the *Stanford-Binet* and may be administered by "teachers as well as other professionals." The instrument consists of one or two items per age level which are at six-month increments. The SIT yields an I.Q. score which has high correlation to the *Stanford-Binet*. Items for all but the very young are given orally and for the most part require oral responses.

> Available from: Western Psychological Services
> 12031 Wilshire Boulevard
> Los Angeles, CA 90025

> Cost: $7.00 Kit (manual, test questions)
> $7.50 Score sheet (package of 100)
> $7.00 Score sheet (2-19 packages)
> $6.50 Score sheet (20+ packages)

Stanford-Binet Intelligence Scale (L. M. Terman, M. A. Merrill, and R. L. Thorndike). Atlanta: Houghton Mifflin, 1972.

> The *Stanford-Binet Intelligence Scale* in its present version (1960) is a result of successive refinements of the original *Binet Scales* developed in France around 1905. As revised, the *Stanford-Binet* is composed of tasks which require a variety of responses from children, including the identification of common objects, hand-eye coordinations, word definition, practical judgments, arithmetic computations, sentence completion, and problem interpretation. As such, the *Stanford-Binet* is based on the assumption that samples of verbal and sensory-motor behavior taken from a child of a given chronological age can serve as an indication of the quality or magnitude of that child's underlying mental ability. The *Stanford-Binet* is suitable for use with children as young as age two and its norms (1960 revision) extend to age eighteen. The intelligence quotient derived from the use of this scale is strongly predictive of academic achievement, particularly during the elementary school years. Thus, many users conceive of the *Stanford-Binet* primarily as a measure of scholastic aptitude. Impressive data in reference to the validity and reliability of this scale have accumulated over the many years of its use.

Available from: Houghton Mifflin Company
666 Miami Circle
N.E.
Atlanta, GA 30324

Cost: $75.00 Examiner's kit (manual, lg. & sm. printed material, miniaturiz-
ed items)
$ 7.50 Record booklets (thirty-five/pkg.)
$ 3.90 Record form (thirty-five/pkg.)

Stanford Early School Achievement Test: Level I or SESAT (R. Madden and E. F.
Gardner). Atlanta: The Psychological Corporation, 1970.

The SESAT measures cognitive abilities upon entrance into kindergarten, at
the end of kindergarten, or upon entrance into first grade. SESAT-I is not a
readiness test except in the sense that a grade three achievement tests is a
readiness measure for grade four. Subtests are: the environment (social and
natural environments, social science, natural science), mathematics
(conservation of number, space, volume; counting; measurement; numera-
tion, classification, simple operations), letters and sounds (upper case letters,
beginning sounds), and aural comprehension (items range from mere recall
to adaptations of aspects of logic). The test is group-administered in five
sessions. Groups of six or seven children per assistant are recommended for
beginning kindergarten students and groups of fifteen per assistant for older
children. Approximate time for administration is ninety minutes. No special
training is needed. Total score and subscore stanines and percentile norms
are available. Split-half reliabilities on the subtests are available. No validity
studies are reported.

Available from: The Psychological Corporation
1372 Peachtree St.
N.E.
Atlanta, GA 30309

Cost: $11.95 thirty-five tests
$ 1.50 Scoring sheet

SRC Language Development Scale. Commack, NY: Suffolk Rehabilitation Center,
1975.

The purpose of the Suffolk Rehabilitation Center *Language Development
Scale* is to determine the receptive and expressive language level of children,
ages birth to six years, and to determine areas of language needing remediation.

A speech pathologist can administer the scale in approximately one-half
hour. The instrument can be given by direct testing, examiner observation of
the child, parent interview, or teacher interview. Usually a combination of
these methods provides the greatest and most accurate information.

Available from: TMA Outreach Program
Suffolk Rehabilitation Center
159 Indian Head Road
Commack, NY 11725

Cost: $ .13

The Teaching Research Placement Test, in *the Teaching Research Curriculum for Moderately and Severely Handicapped* (H. D. Fredricks et al.). Springfield: Charles C. Thomas, 1976.

This criterion-referenced instrument was developed for moderately and severely handicapped children, birth to eight. It has four parts: language skills composed of receptive language skills, reading, expressive language skills and writing skills; self-help skills composed of dressing, eating, toileting, and personal hygiene; cognitive skills composed of personal information concepts, cultural concepts, number concepts, monetary concepts, and telling-time concepts; and motor development skills composed of tone normalization activities, gross motor-basic, gross motor-lower and upper extremity, body orientation, fine motor-lower and upper extremity, strength skills, and recreation skills.

Besides assessment, the instrument provides a means of individualized programming for handicapped children in the designated curriculum areas.

The Teaching Research Curriculum for Moderately and Severely Handicapped is designed to provide a comprehensive list of behaviors that should be taught. It is to be used in a program which designates individual objectives for each child. Tasks are analyzed and sequenced.

Available from: Charles C. Thomas
301-327 E. Lawrence Avenue
Springfield, IL 62717

Cost: $18.50

Test of Basic Experiences or TOBE (M. H. Moss). Monterey: CTB/McGraw-Hill, 1975.

The TOBE indicates how well a child's experiences have prepared him for his introduction to many of the scholastic activities that he will encounter. The TOBE battery is available at Level K for preschool and kindergarten age children, and at Level L for kindergarten and grade one age examinees. Each battery contains five tests: general concepts, mathematics (fundamental concept, relationships, quantitative terms), language (vocabulary, sentence structure, verb tense, sound-symbol relationships, letter recognition, listening skills), science (observations, groups, social roles, customs, safety, human emotions). TOBE is group-administered and paced. It is recommended that one proctor be provided for each four to six children for preschool and kindergarten groups and one for each six to ten children in the first grade. Each test requires about twenty-five minutes to give (125 minutes in all). It is suggested that the five tests be given on five different days. No special training is needed to administer the tests. The tests may be hand scored or a test-scoring service is available if desired. Grade stanine, standard score, and percentile norms are reported for each test. Test-retest reliability studies are in progress. Content validity was studied by use of a validation panel of kindergarten and grade one teachers and the results are reported.

Available from: CTB/McGraw-Hill
Del Monte Research Park
Monterey, CA 93940

Cost: $36.00 Complete battery - level K or L (thirty to a package)

Utah Test of Language Development (M. Meacham, L. Jex, J. D. Jones). Salt Lake City: Communication Research Associates, 1972.

This test is designed to measure expressive and receptive language skills in children nine months through sixteen years.

The test, which is a scale that has been put in test form, is relatively easy to administer and score. From the tally of correct and incorrect responses, the child receives a language age.

There are reliability data. Norms are reported but vary in number from item to item. It takes approximately thirty minutes to administer the test. The examiner must be skilled in eliciting optimum language responses from the child.

Available from: Communication Research Associates
Box 11012
Salt Lake City, UT 84111

Cost: $20.00 Complete kit

Vallett Developmental Survey (R. E. Vallett). Palo Alto: Consulting Psychologists Press, 1966.

This survey helps in evaluating various developmental abilities of children between the ages of two and seven to aid in planning individualized learning programs. It consists of 233 tasks in the areas of motor integration and physical development (seventeen items), tactile discrimination (eleven items), auditory discrimination (thirty-six items), visual-motor coordination (nineteen items), visual discrimination (fifty-three items), language development and verbal fluency (thirty items), and conceptual development (sixty-seven items). The survey is individually administered and paced. Some practice is needed to give the test. Many props, all inexpensive and readily available, are needed. The author considers the survey incomplete by itself and recommends that it be supplemented with measures of family background, prior learning experiences, and subjective estimates of the child's motivation for learning, social judgment, interests, general adaptivity, and common sense. Age norms for each of the tasks are included. No other psychometric data were provided for review.

Available from: Consulting Psychologists Press
577 College Ave.
Palo Alto, CA 94306

Cost: $ 1.25 Specimen set (two booklets & one manual)
$ .75 Manual
$ 3.50 Card set
$ 10.50 Complete kit (ten workbooklets, ten scoring booklets, one manual, one card set)

$ 14.00 Survey sets (pkg. of 25)
$ 52.00   "   (pkg. of 100)
$250.00   "   (pkg. of 500)

The Vane Kindergarten Test (J. R. Vane). Brandon, VT: Clinical Psychology Publishing Co., Inc., 1968.

The Vane Kindergarten Test is a short screening instrument designed to screen for school readiness in vocabulary, perceptual motor, and draw-a-man. The instrument is appropriate for children aged four to six-and-a-half years. It is individually administered by a trained psychologist and takes twenty-five to forty minutes for administration. The vocabulary and perceptual motor portion of the test was standardized on a sample of 1,000 children and the draw-a-man portion on 400 children in a lower-middle-class school district in the Northeastern part of the United States. There is adequate reliability and validity information.

Available from: Clinical Psychology Publishing Co., Inc.
                 4 Conant Sq.
                 Brandon, VT 05733

Cost: $4.00 Manual
      $3.50 Record sheets - fifty to a package

Verbal Language Development Scale (M. J. Meacham). Circle Pines, MN: American Guidance Service, Inc., 1971.

The *Verbal Language Development Scale* is an extension of the communication portion of the *Vineland Social Maturity Scale*. It is an informant interview instrument for children from one month of age to fifteen years. It has the advantage of tapping the child's behavior in familiar settings. There are many items for the younger ages (talks, imitates sounds, uses names of familiar objects) and fewer but more complex descriptions for the older years. Definitions of behavior are given in the manual. Half credit is allowed for behaviors that are in an emerging state. Scores may be converted into a language age, which has been standardized on a sample of 120 normal children. The scale consists of a total of fifty items—six on listening, thirty-one on speaking, five on reading, and eight on writing.

Available from: American Guidance Service, Inc.
                 Publishers Building
                 Circle Pines, MN 55014

Cost: $2.35 twenty-five to a package (1301)
      $ .90 Manual (1302)

Vineland Social Maturity Scale (E. A. Doll). Circle Pines, MN: American Guidance Service, Inc., 1965.

The *Vineland* assesses progress toward social maturity, competence, or independence in subjects from birth to adulthood. Items are designed to elicit factual descriptions of the examinee's habitual or customary behavior as an established mode of conduct. The items are arranged in order of increasing difficulty and represent progressive maturation in self-help, self-direction, locomotion, occupation, communications, and social relations. Detailed descriptions of the behaviors tapped by each item are available. The mean age of expected performance of each behavior for normal subjects by total sample and sex is provided. Total scores may be converted to social ages or social quotients. The scale is scored on the basis of information obtained in an interview with someone intimately familiar with the person scored, or the person himself. The interviewer needs practice and experience in the techniques involved. Illustrative interviews with subjects of various types and ages are available. Test-retest reliabilities, comparisons of social age and social quotients with chronological age, and item validation studies with normal and abnormal populations are reported.

Available from: American Guidance Service, Inc.
Publishers Building
Circle Pines, MN 55014

Cost: $2.90 twenty-five to a package (1231)
$1.90 Manual (1232)

Walker Problem Behavior Identification Checklist (H. M. Walker). Los Angeles: Western Psychological Services, 1970.

This instrument is a quick way to identify children with behavior problems. It consists of fifty items which are checked "present" or "not present" in the particular child. It can be filled out by anyone familiar with the child. The items form five scales: acting-out, withdrawal, distractability, disturbed peer relations, and immaturity. Certain items might be chosen as indicative of a particular problem, of specific interest to a program—e.g. "is listless and continually tired" or "stutters, stammers, or blocks on saying words." Cut-off points for disturbance are included, but norms are given only for grades four, five, and six. Items are appropriate for preschoolers, but centers would probably want to set up their own scoring systems.

Available from: Western Psychological Services
Publishers and Distributors
12031 Wilshire Blvd.
Los Angeles, CA 90025

Cost: $9.50 Kit (100 W-97A Forms and 1 W-97B Manual)
$8.50 1 Pad (100 W-97A Forms)
$7.00 2-19 Pads
$6.00 20+ pads
$2.50 W-97B Manual

Wide Range Achievement Tests (K. F. Jastak and S. R. Jastak). Atlanta: The Psychological Corporation, 1965.

These tests measure achievement in reading, spelling, and arithmetic from preschool through adulthood. Age norms are given for ages five and up. Scores are given in grade equivalents, standard scores, and percentiles. The reading subtest consists of recognizing and naming letters and naming words. The spelling subtest consists of copying marks resembling letters, writing the name, and writing words to dictation. The arithmetic subtest involves counting, reading, number symbols, solving oral problems, and performing written computations. The three subtests take twenty to thirty minutes.

Available from: The Psychological Corporation
1372 Peachtree St.
N.E.
Atlanta, GA 30309

Cost: $5.95 Test booklets (fifty to a package)
$4.90 Manual

Yellow Brick Road (C. Kalestrom). Austin: Learning Concepts, 1975.

The *Yellow Brick Road* is designed to identify children whose patterns of functioning in the motor, visual, auditory, and language areas indicate the need for diagnostic follow-up in a specific area. This instrument may be administered to children 4.9 to 6.9 months. *The Yellow Brick Road* consists of four batteries which are administered on a one-to-one basis in a group setting by trained professionals, paraprofessionals, or volunteers. Each battery contains six subtests with six items per subtest. The children move one at a time along a yellow brick road to play "games" on a one-to-one basis with an operator. The sequence of the batteries allows the child to move from nonverbal, to motor, to visual, to auditory, and finally to language skills. The entire battery takes one hour, with twenty-four children completing the screening every two hours.

Some predictive reliability has been reported. Other technical data will be available by the summer of 1977.

Available from: Learning Concepts
2501 N. LaMar
Austin, TX 78707

Cost: $29.95

The Matrix:
A Guide to
the Instruments
Lee Cross

112

INSTRUMENTS

	Page No.
ABC Inventory	63
Adaptive Behavior Scales	64
Assessment by Behavior Rating	64
Assessment Programming Guide for Infants and Preschoolers	65
Auditory Discrimination Test	65
Basic Concept Inventory	66
Bayley Scales of Infant Development	66
The Bayley Scales of Infant Development Modifications for Youngsters with Handicapped Conditions	67
Beery-Butenica Developmental Test of Visual-Motor Integration	67
Behavioral Developmental Profile	68
Bender Motor Gestalt Test	68
Birth-3 Scale	69
Boehm Test of Basic Concepts	69
Burks Behavior Rating Scales	70
Bzoch-League Receptive-Expressive Emergent Language Scale	70
Cain Levine Social Competency Scale	71
California Preschool Social Competency Scale	71
Callier-Azusa Scales	72
Carolina Developmental Profile	72
Cassel Developmental Record	72

AGE

USE

PERFORMANCE FACTORS

Screening
Diagnostic
Assessment

Language
Perception
Fine Motor
Gross Motor
Social-Emotional
Reasoning
School Readiness

.5
1
1.5
2
2.5
3
3.5
4
4.5
5
5.5
6
6.5
7
7.5
8

114

INSTRUMENTS

	Page No.
Cattell Infant Intelligence Scale	73
Children's Self-Social Constructs Test	73
CIRCUS	74
Classroom Screening	74
Communicative Evaluation Chart	75
Comprehensive Early Education Profile	75
Comprehensive Identification Process	76
Criterion-Referenced Placement Tests	76
Del Rio Language Screening Test	76
Detroit Tests of Learning Aptitude	77
Developmental Indicators for the Assessment of Learning	77
Developmental Profile	78
Developmental Therapy Objective Rating Form	79
The Early Intervention Developmental Profile	79
Eliot-Pearson Screening Profile	80
EMI Assessment Scale	80
Frostig Developmental Test of Visual Perception	81
Fluharty Preschool Language Screening Test	81
The Functional Profile	81
Goldman Fristoe Test of Articulation	82

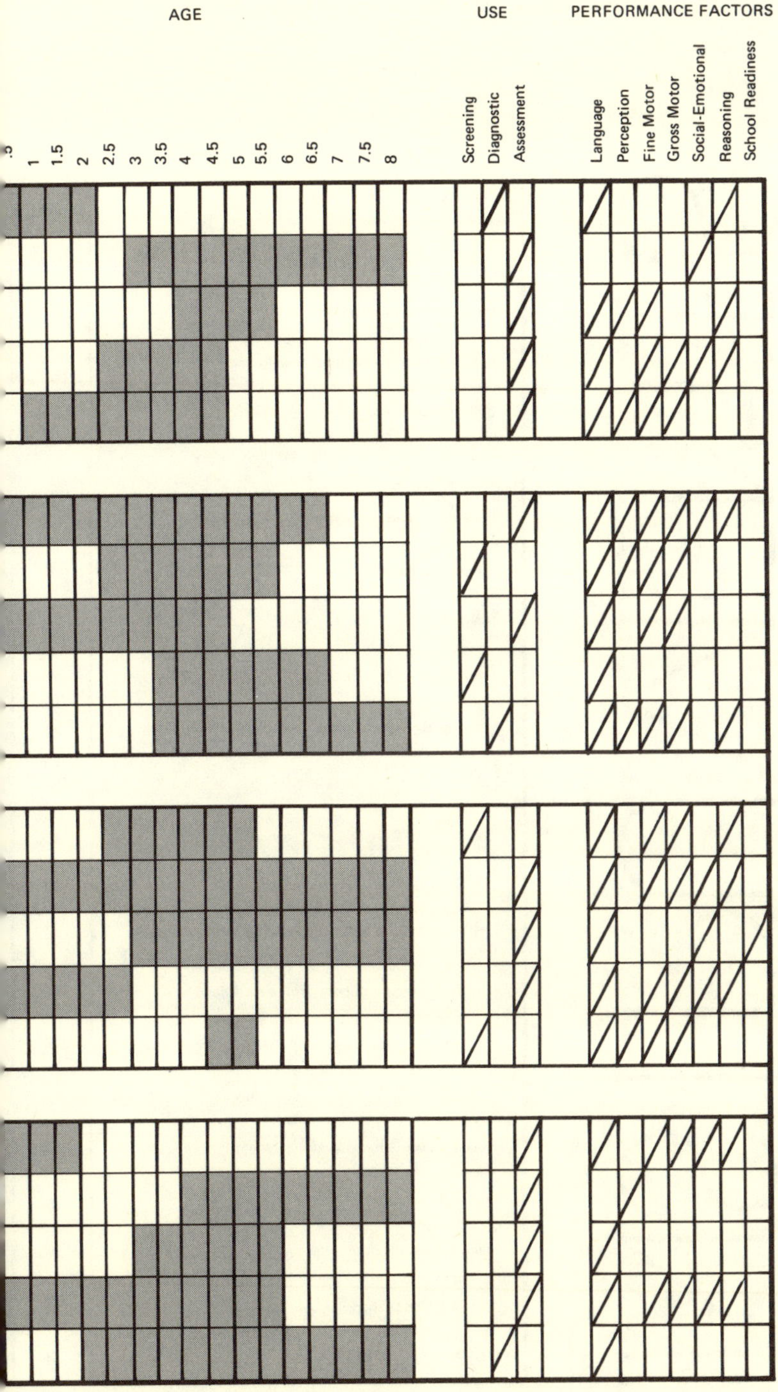
AGE
USE
PERFORMANCE FACTORS
.5
1
1.5
2
2.5
3
3.5
4
4.5
5
5.5
6
6.5
7
7.5
8
Screening
Diagnostic
Assessment
Language
Perception
Fine Motor
Gross Motor
Social-Emotional
Reasoning
School Readiness

INSTRUMENTS

	Page No.
Goldman Fristoe Test of Auditory Discrimination	82
Goodenough Harris Drawing Test	83
Harris Articulation Scale	83
Houston Test for Language Development	83
Illinois Test of Psycholinguistic Ability	84
Individual Child Assessment	84
Infant Evaluation Scale	85
Infant Parent Training Program Checklist	85
Informal Teacher Assessment Instrument	85
Kindergarten Evaluation of Learning Potential	86
Koontz Child Development Program	86
Learning Accomplishment Profile	87
Learning Accomplishment Profile Diagnostic Edition	87
Learning Accomplishment Profile for Infants	88
The Lexington Developmental Scale	88
Marshalltown Behavioral Development Profile	89
McCarthy Scales of Children's Abilities	90
Meeting Street School Screening Test	90
Memphis Comprehensive Development Scales	91
Metropolitan Readiness Tests	91

AGE USE PERFORMANCE FACTORS

.5 1 1.5 2 2.5 3 3.5 4 4.5 5 5.5 6 6.5 7 7.5 8

Screening
Diagnostic
Assessment

Language
Perception
Fine Motor
Gross Motor
Social-Emotional
Reasoning
School Readiness

INSTRUMENTS

	Page No.
Milani-Comparetti Motor Developmental Test	92
Minnesota Preschool Scale	92
Missouri Children's Picture Series	93
Move-Grow-Learn Survey	93
Northwestern Syntax Screening Test	94
Oseretsky Test of Motor Proficiency	94
Peabody Individual Achievement Test	94
Peabody Picture Vocabulary Test	95
Perceptual Skills Curriculum	95
Portage Guide to Early Education	96
Preschool Attainment Record	96
Preschool Inventory	96
Preschool Language Scale	97
Preschool Screening System	97
Primary Mental Abilities	98
The Psychiatric Behavior Scale	98
Pupil Progress Evaluation Plan	99
Referral Form Checklist of Problem Behaviors	99
Scales of Early Communication Skills for Hearing-Impaired Children	100
School Readiness Survey	100

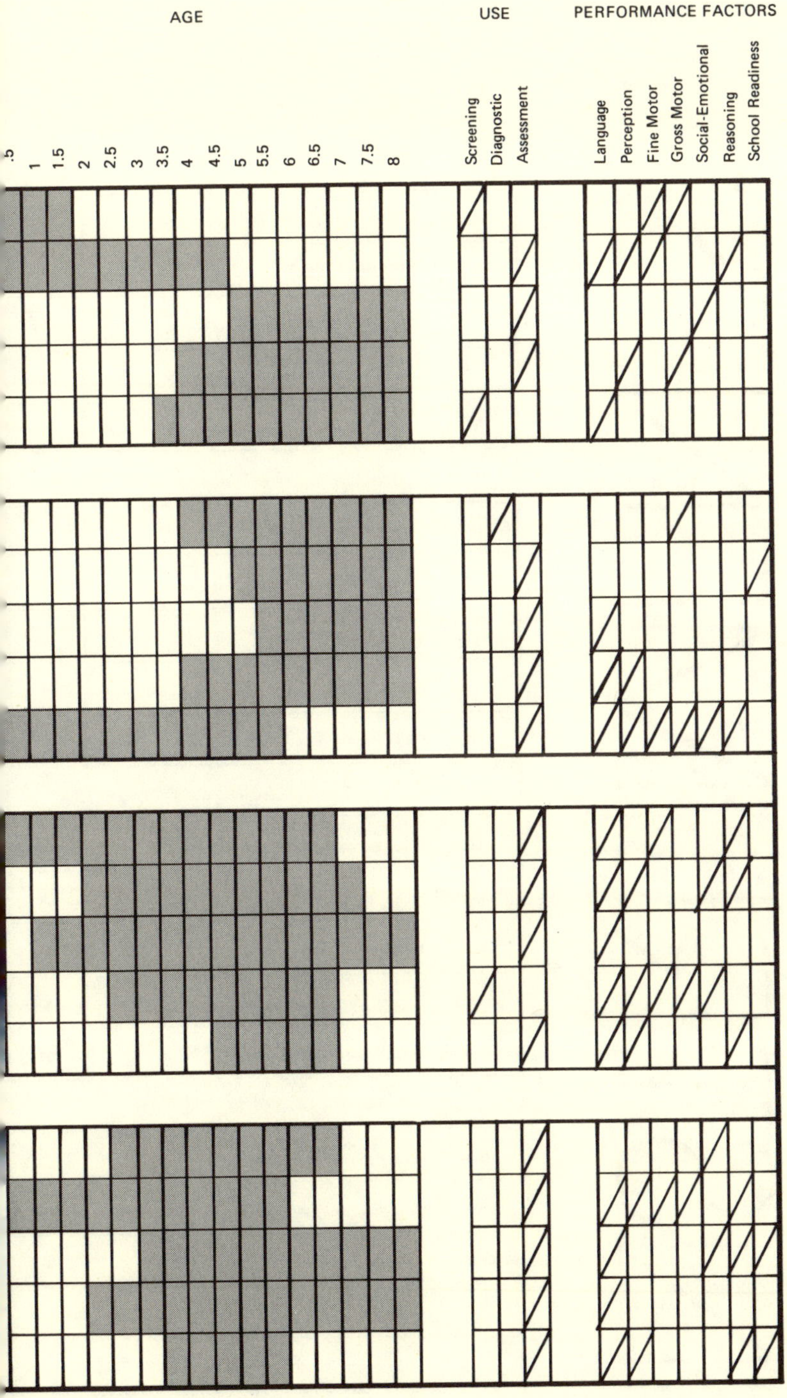
AGE
.5
1
1.5
2
2.5
3
3.5
4
4.5
5
5.5
6
6.5
7
7.5
8
USE
Screening
Diagnostic
Assessment
PERFORMANCE FACTORS
Language
Perception
Fine Motor
Gross Motor
Social-Emotional
Reasoning
School Readiness

INSTRUMENTS

	Page No.
Search and Teach	101
SEEC Developmental Wheel	101
SEED Developmental Profiles	102
SEED Reflex and Therapeutic Evaluation	102
The Slosson Intelligence Test	103
Stanford-Binet Intelligence Scale	103
Stanford Early School Achievement Test	104
SRC Language Development Scale	104
The Teaching Research Placement Test	105
Test of Basic Experiences	105
Utah Test of Language Development	106
Vallett Developmental Survey	106
The Vane Kindergarten Test	107
Verbal Language Development Scale	107
Vineland Social Maturity Scale	107
Walker Problem Behavior Identification Checklist	108
Wide Range Achievement Tests	108
Yellow Brick Road	109

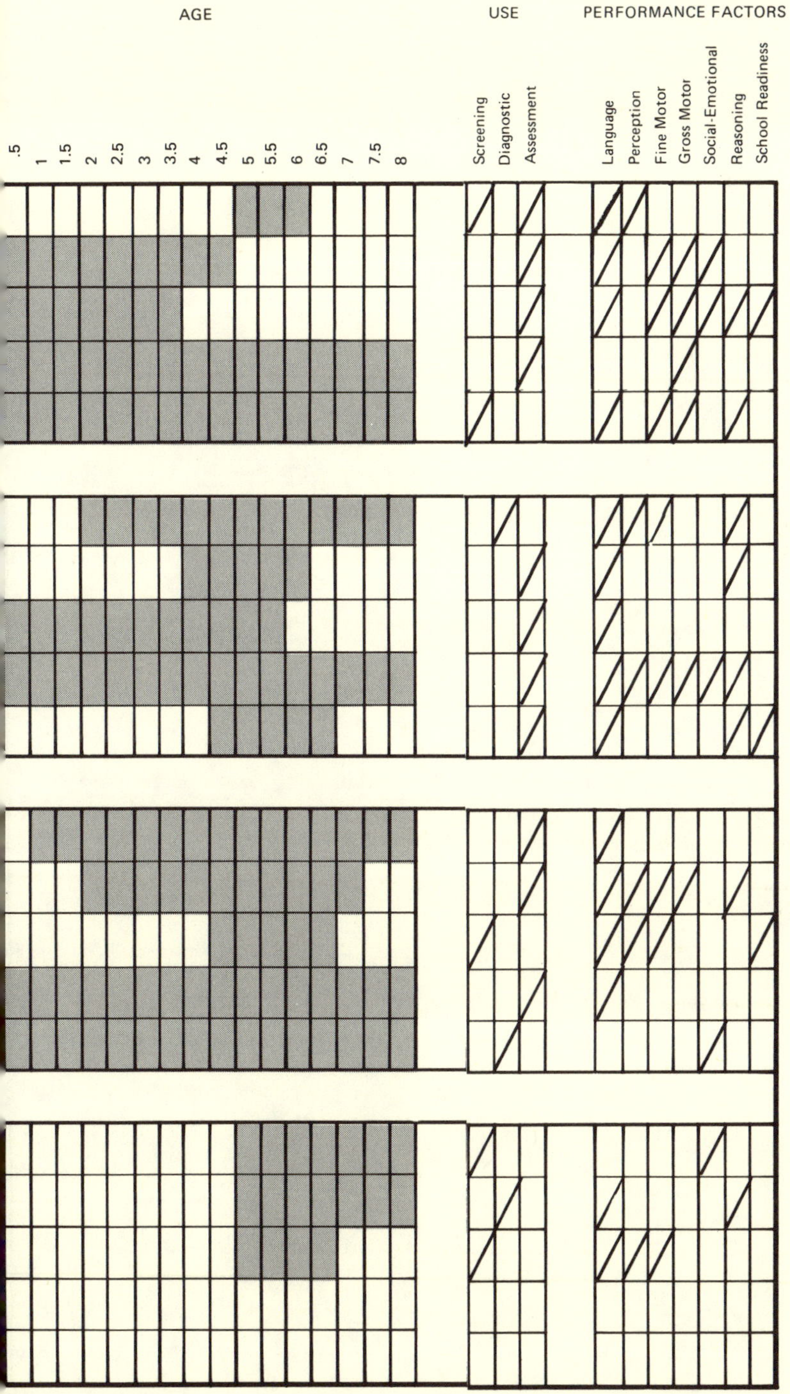
AGE
USE
PERFORMANCE FACTORS
.5
1
1.5
2
2.5
3
3.5
4
4.5
5
5.5
6
6.5
7
7.5
8
Screening
Diagnostic
Assessment
Language
Perception
Fine Motor
Gross Motor
Social-Emotional
Reasoning
School Readiness

Index

ABC Inventory, 24, 63, 112
Adair, N., 63
Adaptive Behavior Scales, 64, 112
Agencies to be contacted, 12
Alpern, G., 78
Alpern-Boll test, 24
American Education Research Association, 31
American Psychological Association, 31
Analysis
    in diagnosis, 26–31
    in evaluation, 53
Anderson, R., 75
Assessment, see Educational assessment
Assessment by Behavior Rating (ABR), 64–65, 112
Assessment-Programming Guide for Infants and Preschoolers, 65, 112
Auditory Discrimination Test, 65–66, 112

Baker, H. J., 77
Bangs, T. E., 42, 69
Barker, W. F., 98
Basic Concept Inventory, 66, 112
Bayley, N., 66
Bayley Scales of Infant Development, 41, 66–67, 112
Modification for Youngsters with Handicapped Conditions, 67, 112
Beery, K., 67
Beery-Buktenica Developmental Test of Visual-motor Integration, 67–68, 112
Behavioral Development Profile, 68, 112
Bender, L., 68
Bender Motor Gestalt Test, 68–69, 112
Birth-3 Scale, 69, 112
Bishop, L., 75
Blesch, G., 63
Bloom, B., 20
Bluma, S., 96
Boehm, A. E., 69
Boehm Test of Basic Concepts or BTBC, 69–70, 112

Bogatz, G., 74
Boll, T., 78
Borneman, A., 98
Brewer, L., 75
Brown, D., 27, 29
Buktenica, N., 67
Burks, H., 70
Burks Behavior Rating Scales, 70, 112
Bzoch, K. P., 70
Bzoch-League Receptive-Expressive Emergent Language Scale, 70, 112

Cain, L. F., 71
Cain Levine Social Competency Scale, 71, 112
Caldwell, B., 19, 96
California Preschool Social Competency Scale or CPSCS, 71–72, 112
Callier-Azusa Scales, 72, 112
Campbell, A. A., 91
Canvass, community, 12–13
Carolina Developmental Profile, 43, 72, 112
Carver, R. P., 41
Case histories, 29–30
Casefinding, 3, 5, 9–15
    definition and purpose of, 4, 9
    screening and, 17–18
Cassel, R. N., 72
Cassel Developmental Record, 72–73, 112
Casto, G., 76
Cattell, P., 73
Cattell Infant Intelligence Scale, 73, 114
Children's Self-Social Constructs Test, 73–74, 114
CIRCUS, 74, 114
Classroom Screening, 74–75, 114
Coleman, C. A., 88
Communicative Evaluation Chart, 75, 114
Community canvass, 12–13
Comprehensive Early Education Profile, 75, 114
Comprehensive Identification Process, 76, 114
Confidential information, 56

Cox, R. C., 41
Criterion-referenced devices, 41–44
Criterion-Referenced Placement
  Tests, 76, 114

Davis, Q. I., 75
Decision-making, definition of, 53
Del Rio Language Screening, 76–77,
  114
Denver Developmental Screening
  Test, 24
Detroit Tests of Learning Aptitude, 77,
  114
D'Eugenio, D. B., 79
Developmental Diagnosis, 41
Developmental Indicators for the As-
  sessment of Learning (DIAL), 24,
  77–78, 114
Developmental Profile, 78, 114
Developmental Sentence Analysis,
  40–41
Developmental Therapy Objective
  Rating Form or DTORF, 78–79, 114
Diagnosis, 3, 5, 25–34
    definition and purpose of, 6–8, 25
Diagnosis
    screening and, 25–26
Dickerson, J., 99
Doll, E. A., 94, 96, 107
Donahue, M., 68, 89
Draper, T., 74
Drezek, W., 85
Dunn, L. M., 94, 95

Early intervention, 19–20, 22
Early Intervention Developmental Pro-
  file and Developmental Screening
  of Handicapped Infants, 79–80, 114
Educational assessment, 3, 5, 35–51
    definition and purpose of, 8, 35
Elder, W. B., 80
Eliot-Pearson Screening Profile, 80,
  114
Elzey, F. F., 71
EMI Assessment Scale, 80, 114
Engelmann, S., 66
Evaluation, see Program evaluation
Evanson, M., 99

Flamer, G. B., 85
Fluharty Preschool Language Screening Test, 81, 114

Foster, R., 64
Fredricks, H. D., 105
Fristoe, M., 82
Frohman, A., 96
Frostig, M., 81
Frostig Developmental Test of Visual
  Perception, 81, 114
Functional Profile, 81–82, 114
Fvatt, R. L., 97

Gallagher, J., 29, 31, 55
Gardner, E. F., 104
Garrett, S., 69
Geers, A. V., 100
Gesell, A., 41
Giessman, N., 74
Gingold, P., 85
Gingold, W., 85
Goldenberg, D., 77
Goldman, R., 82
Goldman Fristoe Test of Articulation,
  82, 114
Goldman Friscoe Woodcock Test of
  Auditory Discrimination, 82, 116
Goodenough, F., 83, 92
Goodenough Harris Drawing Test, 83,
  116
Gordon, T., 19
Griffen, P.M., 87, 88
Griffiths, N., 91

Hagin, R., 101
Hailey, J., 84
Hainsworth, M., 97
Hainsworth, P., 90, 97
Hallahan, D., 27
Harris, D., 83
Harris, G. S., 83
Harris Articulation Scale, 83, 116
Hauessermann, E., 29, 38
Henderson, E., 73
Hering, S., 74, 84
Herset, J., 102
Hildreth, G., 91
Hilliard, J., 96
Hoffman, H., 67
Houston Test for Language Develop-
  ment, 83–84, 116
Huestis, L. L., 93
Humphreys, F., 98
Hunt, J. McV., 48

Illinois Test of Psycholinguistic Ability, 40, 84, 116
Individual Child Assessment, 84, 116
Infant Evaluation Scale, 85, 116
Infant-Parent Training Program Checklist, 85, 116
Informal Teacher Assessment Instrument, 85–86, 116
Interview, screening, 29
Investigation, typical areas of, 28
Irwin, J., 88
Issacson, S., 74

Jastak, K. F., 108
Jastak, S. R., 108
Jex, L., 106
Jones, J. D., 106
Jordan, F. L., 100
Jorgensen, E., 102
Jorgenson, G., 102
Joyner, L., 75
Jungeblut, A., 74

Kalestrom, C., 109
Kaufman, J., 27
Keiser, A., 68
Kindergarten Evaluation of Learning Potential or KELP, 86, 116
King, K. F., 75
Kirk, S., 84
Kirk, W., 84
Knight, G., 98
Koontz, C., 86
Koontz Child Developmental Program:
Training Activities for the First 48 Months, 86–87, 116

Lavatelli, C. S., 48
League, R., 70
Learning Accomplishment Profile, 87, 116
Learning Accomplishment Profile-Diagnostic Edition (LAP-D), 87–88, 116
Learning Accomplishment Profile for Infants: Experimental Edition, 88, 116
Lee, L., 94
Leland, B., 77
Leland, H., 64
Leverman, D., 76

Levine, S., 71
Lewis, M., 71
Lexington Developmental Scale, 88–89, 116
Lillie, D., 19
Little, D. L., 72
Little, T. L., 91
Location of children, 10–11, 13–14
Long, B., 73

Madden, R., 104
Mardell, C., 77
Markwardt, F., 94
Marshalltown Behavioral Development Profile, 89, 116
Massey, J., 100
Matheny, P., 75
McCarthy, D., 90
McCarthy, J., 84
McCarthy Scales of Children's Abilities, 90, 116
McGauvran, M., 91
Meacham, M., 106, 107
Meeting Street School Screening Test (MSSST), 90, 116
Meisells, S. J., 80
Memphis Comprehensive Development Scales, 91, 116
Meredith, M., 75
Merrill, M. A., 103
Metropolitan Readiness Tests, 91–92, 116
Milani-Comparetti Development Test, 92, 118
Miles, M., 75
Minnesota Preschool Scale, 92, 118
Missouri Children's Picture Series, 93, 118
Montgomery, J., 68, 89
Mood cues, 46
Moog, J. S., 100
Moss, M. H., 105
Move-Grow-Learn Survey, 93–94, 118

Newquist, J., 75
Nihira, N., 64
Norm-referenced devices, 40–41
Northwestern Syntax Screening Test, 94, 118

Observation
    assessment, 44–47
    screening, 29
Ordinal Scales of Psychological De-
    velopment, 48
Orpet, R. E., 93
Oseretsky Test of Motor Proficiency,
    94, 118

Pallam, S., 102
Palmer, J., 29
Pauker, J., 93
Paulson, C., 53
Peabody Individual Achievement Test,
    94–95, 118
Peabody Picture Vocabulary Test or
    PPVT, 95, 118
Pearson, P., 92
Perceptual Skills Curriculum, 95–96,
    118
Piagetian devices, 38, 47–48
Pollan, P., 102
Portage Guide to Early Education, 96,
    118
Preschool Attainment Record, 96, 118
Preschool Inventory, 42, 96–97, 118
Preschool Language Scale, 97, 118
Preschool Screening System (PSS),
    97–98, 118
Primary Mental Abilities, 98, 118
Program evaluation, 3, 5, 53–58
    definition and purpose of, 8, 53
    formative vs. summative, 54
Psychiatric Behavior Scale, 98–99,
    118
Public awareness activities, 11–12
Pupil Progress Evaluation Plan, 99,
    118

Quick, A. P., 91

Referral Form Checklist of Problem
    Behaviors, 99–100, 118
Rice, L., 92
Risan, S., 98
Robeck, M. C., 83
Roecker, V., 68
Rogers, S., 79
Rosner, J., 95

Sadler, L., 98
Sanford, A. R., 41, 87, 88

Scales of Early Communication Skills
    for Hearing-Impaired Children, 100,
    118
Scarvia, A., 74
School Readiness or SRS, 100–1, 118
Screening, 3, 5, 17–24
    casefinding and, 17–18
    definition and purpose of, 4–6, 17
    diagnosis and, 25–26
Search and Teach, 101, 120
Sedwell, G., 74
SEEC Developmental Wheel, 101–2,
    120
SEED Developmental Profile, 102, 120
SEED Reflex and Therapeutic Evalua-
    tion, 102–3, 120
Sharp, E., 64
Shearer, M., 96
Shellhas, M., 64
Silver, A., 101
Simeonsson, R., 27n
Sines, J., 93
Sines, L., 93
Siqueland, E. M., 90
Skills to be assessed, 35–36
Slosson, R. L., 103
Slosson Intelligence Test, 103, 120
Smiley, C., 82
Smith, L., 68
Smith, M., 75
Spurlock, L., 99
SRC Language Development Scale,
    104, 120
Standardization of measurement in-
    struments, 22–23, 29
Standards, definition of, 53
Standards for Educational and Psy-
    chological Tests, 31
Stanford-Binet Intelligence Scale,
    103–4, 120
Stanford Early School Achievement,
    104, 120
Steiner, U. G., 97
Stillman, R., 72
Stoke, R. E., 55
Stufflebeam, O. L., 55
Swanson, J. E., 101
Synthesis in diagnosis, 26, 31–32

Tarchin, C., 74
Target population, 9–10
Teaching Research Placement Test, 105, 120

Terman, L. M., 103
Test of Basic Experiences or TUBE,
  105–6, 120
Thompson, A., 75
Thorndike, R. L., 103
Thurstone, T. G., 98
Toronto, A., 76
Trembath, J., 92

Umansky, W., 65
Utah Test of Language Development,
  106, 120
Uzgiris, I. C., 48

Vallett, R. E., 106, 120
Vallett Developmental Survey, 106–7,
  120
Vane, J. R., 107
Vane Kindergarten Test, 107, 120
Verbal Language Development Scale,
  107, 120
Vineland Social Maturity Scale,
  107–8, 120

Walker, H. M., 108
Walker Problem Behavior Identifica-
  tion Checklist, 108, 120
Ward, W., 74
Weiss, R., 81
Wepman, J., 65
Wide Range Achievement Tests,
  108–9, 120
Wiegerink, R., 27n
Wilson, D. C., 87
Wilson, J. A. R., 86
Wiske, M. S., 80
Wolfe, S., 102
Wood, M. M., 78, 99
Woodcock, R., 82

Yates, A., 74
Yellow Brick Road, 109, 120

Zehrbach, R. R., 76
Ziller, R., 73
Zimmerman, I. L., 97